骨科英文写作实用教程

主　编　郭炯炯

副主编　刘国栋

苏 州 大 学 出 版 社

图书在版编目(CIP)数据

骨科英文写作实用教程/郭炯炯主编. —苏州：
苏州大学出版社, 2020.12
ISBN 978-7-5672-3436-9

Ⅰ.①骨… Ⅱ.①郭… Ⅲ.①骨科学-英语-写作-
教材 Ⅳ.①R68

中国版本图书馆 CIP 数据核字(2020)第 263608 号

书　　名：骨科英文写作实用教程
主　　编：郭炯炯
责任编辑：周建国
助理编辑：万才兰
封面设计：刘　俊

出版发行：苏州大学出版社(Soochow University Press)
地　　址：苏州市十梓街1号　邮编：215006
印　　装：苏州工业园区美柯乐制版印务有限责任公司
网　　址：http://www.sudapress.com
邮　　箱：sdcbs@suda.edu.cn
邮购热线：0512-67480030
销售热线：0512-67481020

开　　本：700mm×1 000mm　1/16　印张：12.25　字数：207 千
版　　次：2020 年 12 月第 1 版
印　　次：2020 年 12 月第 1 次印刷
书　　号：ISBN 978-7-5672-3436-9
定　　价：45.00 元

凡购本社图书发现印装错误,请与本社联系调换。服务热线:0512-67481020

《骨科英文写作实用教程》
编　委　会

目录

第一章

概 论

1.1 英文论文的重要性

随着中国的国际影响力越来越大,中国医学界的实力也日益壮大。中国医学界走向世界并影响世界的一个重要指标就是医疗行业从业者在高水平期刊上发表高水平论文。发表论文可以向外界介绍自己的研究成果、临床发现和学术思想。现今,大多数论文在高水平期刊上是用英文发表的。因此,医疗行业从业者能够写出合格甚至优秀的英文论文就显得尤为重要。

如今,多数高校不仅注重学生对理论内容的学习,还对学生的实践及科研能力提出了要求,而论文的撰写和发表就是其中一个重要指标。在撰写和发表论文的过程中,学生会查阅大量国内外文献,经过研究后形成一套科学的逻辑思维体系,可以为以后工作或进一步深造夯实基础。因此,对本科生及研究生的英文论文写作能力的培养也应被提上各高校的日程。

在科研方面,取得成果后应尽快发表英文论文,这样可以使自己的工作成果为本领域的国内外同行所知晓,进而使自己为同行所熟知,并获得分享国际学术资源的资格,如受邀参加国际会议、参编专著、到国际高水平实验室或大学做访问学者等,为进一步研究奠定基础。由此可见,发表英文论文是成长为具有国际学术影响力的医学研究者的重要一步。此外,医学研究者及时发表自己的研究成果能够为从事相关研究的同行提供有价值的参考信息,便于他们根据最新的研究进展及时对正在进行的相关研究做出必要的调整,从而推动相关研究方向的学术发展。

1.2 英文论文的分类

针对骨科医学学生在专业英语表达实践中遇到的困难,本书试图给他们提供一些英文论文写作方法。下面先简单介绍英文论文的分类。

英文论文种类繁多,但主要分为以下七类。

(1) 论著类

论著类论文又名原著,是各类医学期刊的核心内容,是报告基础、临床、预防等探究成果和实践经验的学术性论文,也是医学生最先要学会、精通的论文类型。把握论著类论文的基本特征和撰写规范后,医学生对其他种类的医学论文的写作也可以触类旁通。

(2) 综述类

综述类论文是研究者就具体专业领域甚至具体研究方向的海量文献进行详尽查阅、分析、科学归纳、客观评述而产生的学术性文章。此类论文可以反映具体学科甚至研究方向当前的最新进展、学术见解等。综述类论文的实用价值一般较高。其撰写内容要点包括确定问题、检索文献、评估文献、总结归纳证据和解释结果。

(3) 病例报告类

病例报告类论文是医学期刊中常见的一个固定栏目内发表的论文类型,主要是分享案例少又典型的病例经验,对特殊病例进行详细记录和描述,试图提供第一手病例的相关资料,具有较高的临床价值。

(4) 述评类

述评类论文是一种具有评论性质的文献类型,是医学期刊不可缺少的组成部分。其作者往往针对某一项目或专题,深入分析发展现状,并对其进行较为全面的评论,评价其理论意义和实践意义,剖析问题并提出自己的观点或建议。此类论文要求观点鲜明、针对性强,其作者多为相关领域的专家。

(5) 简报类

简报类论文一般以摘要或简报的形式发表,其全文可在其他期刊继续发表。

（6）会议纪要类

会议纪要是一种常见的报告形式，包括世界性的编委会会议纪要和学术会议纪要，要求简明扼要、准确反映主题。

（7）消息类

消息类论文的内容涵盖全球学术动态、医学新闻、科研简讯、会议预告等，强调时效性，要求简短，表达要完整清楚，不能模棱两可。

这几种主要的论文形式中，论著类和综述类是最基本的两种类型。本书以具体文献为例来讲述骨科英文论文的写作，重点介绍论著类骨科英文论文的基本写作方法和技巧。

1.3 英文论文的撰写

思路清晰是写好骨科英文论文的基本条件，我们对研究领域、研究成果及其意义要有清楚的了解。另外，英文写作能力也极其重要，我们需要熟练运用正确的语法及词汇来组织完整的句子和段落。论文要逐字逐句慢慢写，这是一个需要下功夫的过程。文中的词句及数据结果的阐述一般都需要经过多次修改才能令人满意。

以下几个论文撰写步骤可供参考。

① 查阅相关研究文献，了解论文的格式、研究领域的前沿及当前面临的问题等。

② 撰写材料与方法和结果部分。这两部分一般是研究者最熟悉的内容，也是一篇论文的核心。需要注意的是，方法与结果要互相匹配，要避免遗漏或多余。

③ 撰写前言部分。完成材料与方法和结果部分的撰写后，写作者对研究的成果、意义、创新点会有更好的阐述，比较容易完成前言部分的撰写。

④ 撰写讨论部分。讨论部分应与前言部分有关联性，都应涉及文献综述和研究成果。

⑤ 撰写结论和摘要部分。结论和摘要是对论文的总结，完成论文主体的撰写后，结论部分和摘要部分一般比较容易撰写。此外，不是每篇论文都一定要有结论部分。

⑥ 拟定标题，撰写致谢及参考文献部分。

⑦ 对论文进行反复修改。

第二章

语言表达技巧

　　文字是用来记载和传播信息的,读者理解的文字中传播的信息与作者希望传达的信息完全一致是语言表达的完美形态。英文的表达包括词汇的选择、语法的应用、标点符号的使用等。在骨科英文论文的撰写中,语言的表达要做到确切、清楚、直接、易懂及精练。做到这几点,英文论文的撰写将不再困难。清晰、准确的表达又是论文写作的重中之重。

　　(1) 确切

　　确切是指在撰写骨科英文论文时,写作者要选择合适的词汇,避免使用意义不确定的词汇,因为用非母语写作时往往会错误使用近义词等。同时,语言的准确并非要求列出所有的内容,而是要选择必要的内容。

　　(2) 清楚

　　清楚是指要避免表意不清。写作者在进行骨科英文写作时往往会写出模棱两可的语句,这会使整篇论文的质量受到影响。表意清楚要做到:避免不必要的复杂表述,包括不必要的复杂词汇和复杂句子;避免产生歧义,包括因单词、语法及标点符号使用不当而造成的歧义。

　　(3) 直接

　　直接是指写作要坦率、直截了当。写作的最终目的是告知,不需要“躲躲藏藏”。撰写论文时,写作者要注意句子语气的把握,并选择醒目、明确的动名词,从而让读者一眼就知道写作者的表意及态度。

（4）易懂

易懂是指易于读者理解。在进行骨科英文论文写作时，写作者常常会使用大量的专业术语，但非医学专业的读者对这些术语不熟悉，阅读时会一头雾水。所以我们在写作时最好能对一些专业术语进行适当的解释。

（5）精练

精练是指避免使用不必要的冗长字句。撰写论文时，我们要学会去除冗长字句，剔除无价值的文字，以及精简长句。

2.1 语法

语法是语言的规则，准确地应用语法才能写出被读者准确理解的文章。对于论文写作者来说，掌握基本的语法规则是不成问题的，但即使是最有经验的写作者，有时也不可避免犯语法错误。因此，语法需要我们尤为注意。

（1）主谓一致

英文中名词有单数、复数，动词也有单数、复数形式，二者要保持一致。主语是单数，谓语动词就用单数；主语是复数，谓语动词就用复数。例如：

① The comedic repertoire of the average anaesthetist needs to be revised in the light of these data. （单数形式）

② Some senders of spam journal invitations are bad eggs, who misrepresent their locations and are usually open access publishers. （复数形式）

none, some, all 作主语时，谓语动词既可以用单数也可以用复数。当 none 与 of 连用时，of 后面的单词是单数时，谓语动词用单数；of 后面的单词是复数时，谓语动词用复数。例如：

① None of the fluid was wasted.

② None of the patients were infected.

表示数量、质量、时间等的词汇作主语时，谓语动词用单数，但如果表示分次添加或减少的数量则用复数。例如：

① 20 g was added.

② 10 g were added stepwise.

（2）强调句式

在英文论文写作中，若要强调某件事情，可以把它放在句首，突出其重要性。例如：

① Before the tsunami arrived, most of the people had moved out. (强调海啸到来之前)

② Most of the people had moved out before the tsunami arrived. (强调搬走)

（3）时态

英文论文基本上用两种时态,即现在时和过去时,偶尔会用到完成时。论文中的时态有它特定的意义,表述已发表的研究成果用现在时,表述未发表的实验和研究结果用过去时,因为还没有得到承认,并且是写论文之前做的事情。一般来说,摘要、材料与方法、结果部分的表达用过去时,而讨论部分则需要交替使用现在时和过去时。例如:

① Platelet-rich plasma (PRP) represents a biological treatment for various musculoskeletal injuries involving tendons, ligaments, cartilage and bone.

② We defined exposure to a specific anesthesia type by one or more charge codes for general or regional anesthesia generated on the day of surgery.

（4）连接词和副词

论文要表达一个完整的思维过程,句子之间的衔接和关系十分重要。句子可以通过连接词、短句或一个整句衔接,衔接的作用就是使前后连贯起来,从而达到说明、推理、讨论的目的。连接词和副词一般可表示因果关系、同等关系、相反关系、相似关系、举例等。例如:

① Nevertheless, the accuracy of self-reported weight has been shown to be inversely related to changes in weight and when weight is changing quickly it may not be reliable. (相反关系)

② Furthermore, trading or rental of licence plates on the secondary market has occurred. (同等关系)

③ For example, Bell et al. found that acquiring a motorised vehicle (motorcycle or car) was associated with a 1.8 kg weight gain in a Chinese sample. (举例)

④ Consequently, the training an undergraduate receives is highly dependent on the motivation, ability, knowledge, and personality of the junior mentor. (因果关系)

⑤ Similarly, elevated CO_2 only enhances N_2 fixation when other nutrients, such as phosphorus and potassium, are added. (相似关系)

（5）冠词

不同于汉语，使用冠词是英语的一大语言特点。因此，我们在撰写英文论文时，要熟练掌握定冠词 the 和不定冠词 a, an 的用法，避免因掌握不熟练而出现漏用。例如：

① The different levels of DNMT3A expression had no effect on the DNA methylation of key regulatory regions of Oct-4.

② This results in an aberrant gene expression profile in many kinds of cancer.

2.2 常见的句子错误

（1）结构不完整

句子缺乏必要的成分，如主语、谓语、宾语等，不符合语法规范。例如：

误：By utilizing population based data to find that tranexamic acid was effective in reducing the need for blood transfusions while not increasing the risk of complications, including thromboembolic events and renal failure.

正：Utilizing population based data, we found that tranexamic acid was effective in reducing the need for blood transfusions while not increasing the risk of complications, including thromboembolic events and renal failure.

（2）句式杂糅

不同的句法结构若置于同等的位置会造成语句结构混乱、语义不清。例如：

误：Electronic medical records were used to evaluate complications and compared with readmission.

正：Complications were evaluated by using electronic medical records and compared with readmission.

（3）主谓不一致

句子主语与谓语不一致，尤其在定语从句与动名词短语的使用中。例如：

误：About a quarter of all the injuries are overuse injuries, which is more likely to occur in non-contact sports.

正：About a quarter of all the injuries are overuse injuries, which are more likely to occur in non-contact sports.

（4）否定结构错误

句子否定结构的错误使用可能带来表意的偏差。例如：

误：Although there is not consensus on a standard threshold to consider as an acceptable balance，a standardized difference of less than 10% or 0.1 to indicate negligible differences between groups has been suggested.

正：Although there is no consensus on a standard threshold to consider as an acceptable balance，a standardized difference of less than 10% or 0.1 to indicate negligible differences between groups has been suggested.

（5）省略不当

在一定语境下，某些句子成分可以省略，但如果错误省略句子成分则会产生语法错误。例如：

误：The expression of DNMT3A in HPV-negative cervical cancer cells（C-33A）was higher than in HPV-positive cervical cancer cells.

正：The expression of DNMT3A in HPV-negative cervical cancer cells（C-33A）was higher than that in HPV-positive cervical cancer cells.

2.3　标点符号的使用

标点符号的正确使用是语言准确表达的重要内容，可以帮助读者更好地理解语句，从而更加明确论文的具体内容。英文论文写作中经常使用的标点符号有逗号、句号、分号、冒号、破折号、连词符、引号等，而感叹号几乎不会被使用。注意，英文中句号为实点（.），没有顿号（、），一般由逗号（,）代替。

写作中应尽量少用不必要的逗号，逗号的频繁使用会增加读者阅读的难度。逗号的使用情况一般包括：状语短语位于句首时，后面跟逗号；句子的并列成分之间用逗号；陈述多条目时，使用逗号分开；状语从句在主句之前时，之间用逗号；在非限制性定语从句之前用逗号。

句号（.）是英文写作中最常用的标点符号，表示一句话结束后的停顿，写作中应避免因滥用而导致表达不流畅。

分号（;）的作用介于句号与逗号之间，分开的两部分关系不如用逗号紧密，又不像句号那样完全分开。英文论文中分号的使用情况包括：关系密切的并列分句之间用分号；数个长的并列词组或分句之间用分号。

冒号（:）是表示补充的标点符号，可吸引读者注意下面的内容。冒号的使用情况包括：列出例子，解释说明词句；下定义或对内容进行介绍、阐释。

破折号(——)用于解释说明前文或做补充说明,表示承接关系。对破折号的使用要谨慎,避免造成语句的不连贯,使用时要与连词符"-"区分。

连词符(-)是医学英文论文写作中较常见的一个符号,可把两个及以上的单词连接起来成为新的合成词。

论文研读

英文论文

Comparison of clinical and patient-reported outcomes of three procedures for recurrent anterior shoulder instability: arthroscopic Bankart repair, capsular shift, and open Latarjet

Yingjie Xu, Kailun Wu, Qianli Ma, Lei Zhang, Yong Zhang, Wu Xu, Jiongjiong Guo

Abstract

Background Best surgical of recurrent anterior shoulder instability remained controversial. We knew little about the superiority and choice between traditional open and modern arthroscopic techniques. We hypothesized that outcomes of all patients will be similar regardless of surgical technique.

Methods A retrospective case-cohort analysis of 168 patients who had recurrent anterior shoulder instability was conducted from September 2010 to December 2013. All cases [mean age 30.8 (range 18 – 50) years] were performed with arthroscopic Bankart repair (33 males/20 females), open Latarjet (34 males/18 females), and capsular shift (31 males/14 females). The average follow-up was 67.6 months (range 60 – 72). The shoulder instability severity index score (ISIS) was more than 3 with an average of 6.4.

Results All treatments proved to be effective in improving shoulder functional status and reducing symptoms, while open Latarjet had an advantage over subjective perception. The Rowe scores in arthroscopic Bankart, open Latarjet, and capsular shift group were 92.3 ± 1.5, 96.2 ± 2.1, and 93.2 ± 2.3, respectively, with significant difference. There was no significant difference in other functional outcomes. However, the open Latarjet group in subjective results [subjective shoulder value (SSV) and subjective shoulder value for sport practice (SSV Sport)] was superior to the others ($P < 0.05$). There were two relapsed cases in arthroscopic Bankart and capsular shift group, respectively, and no recurrence in open Latarjet group.

Conclusions Arthroscopic Bankart repair has the advantage of mini-invasion and rapid recovery. Capsular shift offers stabilizing of inferior or multidirectional type, especially for little bone defect. Latarjet was more effective in reducing recurrence with higher stability.

Level of evidence Therapeutic level III

Keywords Shoulder, Instability, Bankart, Latarjet, Capsular shift

Introduction

Recurrent anterior shoulder instability may be caused by avulsion of the anterior glenoid rim and irreversible stretching of anteroinferior capsule, which is known as a Bankart lesion. It has been reported that the incidence is up to 60% with increasing trend. The optimal surgical treatment of recurrent anterior shoulder instability associated with severe glenoid defects and capsular deficiency remains challenging. It was a disabling condition commonly treated with arthroscopic Bankart repair, open Latarjet, or capsular shift.

With the development of arthroscopy, Bankart repair has been currently the preferred choice to treat recurrent instability with nearly 90% of surgeons accepted. Several studies have shown that Bankart repair ensured greater stability and less recurrence compared with the others. However, opponents held that there were unmeasured confounding factors, which were probably related to differences in outcome, including sex, age, hyperlaxity, history of instability, level of sports, and lesions of glenoid and humeral bone. In addition, the recurrence of these techniques varied obviously in the literature. They believed that surgical procedure should focus more on anatomic repairs, which Bankart repair may not. Today, we all knew that glenohumeral bone loss and capsular deficiency were considered to remain ubiquitous in anterior shoulder instability. It was known as Broca-Perthes-Bankart (a combination of capsular laxity and glenohumeral ligament avulsion). The Latarjet procedure has been shown to be a reliable technique which fixed the failings of Bankart repair and had a lower rate of recurrent instability. Furthermore, the capsular shift was widely used in the USA because it rectified both the Bankart lesion and capsular laxity. These three procedures have become mainstream for recurrent anterior shoulder instability. Nevertheless, we did not have enough knowledge about the superiority between traditional open and modern arthroscopic techniques according to available findings. There was still no rational proposal so that the choice of treatments often depended on training or preferences of a surgeon.

It was very important for surgeons to acquire associated knowledge about Bankart and open surgery, which can provide accurate preoperative references of the risks and benefits. In this study, we evaluated the three treatments with a larger sample size and longer follow-up (at least 36 months). The aim of this study was to assess the functional and subjective results of these surgical and determine which one better suited our needs.

Materials and methods

Patients

Between September 2010 and December 2013, we performed a retrospective study to analyze the outcomes of recurrent anterior shoulder instability at our hospital. This study plan was approved by the local ethics committee, and the consent was obtained.

All patients had a diagnosis of recurrent anterior shoulder instability as the main symptom, who had dislocation of the shoulder joint with slight external force, for at least 1 year. In the meantime, we screened a random sample of subjects of 18 – 50 age group. Other inclusion criteria were subjects with a score of at least 3 on the instability severity index score (ISIS), higher sports requirement (especially over-shoulder movement). Exclusion criteria included a condition other than osteoarthritis of the shoulder (significant changes in joint space), multiple recurrent shoulder subluxation or dislocation, first dislocated, severe epilepsy, unclosed osteoepiphysis, severe glenoid bone loss (glenoid loss of contour on anteroposterior radiograph), an active infection, and a major medical illness. Eventually, 168 patients met the above-defined criteria. Until now, 18 patients had incomplete data, leaving a cohort of 150 patients [mean age 30.8 (range 18 – 50) years, 100 right shoulders, mean ISIS 6.4] available for review at a minimum of 36 months. From these patients, three groups have been selected according to different surgical procedures (Bankart repair, Latarjet procedure, and capsular shift). Demographic data and preoperative characteristics had no statistical difference among the three groups (Table 1).

Table 1　Demographic data and preoperative characteristics

Variable	Bankart ($n = 53$)	Latarjet ($n = 52$)	Capsular shift ($n = 45$)
Age (years, mean ± SD)	29.81 ± 4.31	31.23 ± 6.12	30.75 ± 3.85
Male/Female	33/20	34/18	31/14
Dominant involvement	37	32	31
Course of preoperative dislocation (months, mean ± SD)	14.25 ± 5.10	13.80 ± 3.13	13.42 ± 3.72
Competitive sport before instability (%)	26 (49.1%)	20 (38.5%)	24 (53.3%)
Hyperlaxity (ER > 85°)(%)	27 (51.0%)	24 (46.2%)	21 (46.7%)
Rowe score(mean ± SD)	48.74 ± 12.08	42.23 ± 14.20	50.87 ± 9.61
ISIS (mean ± SD)	6.16 ± 2.81	7.01 ± 3.02	6.50 ± 2.56

ER external rotation; *ISIS* instability severity index score. Competitive sport: ball games, throwing events, gymnastics, and so on. $P < 0.05$ was considered statistically significant.

Latarjet procedure should be considered as the first choice if the loss of the anterior glenoid rim was larger than 50% of the maximum anteroposterior diameter of glenoid on routine computed tomography (CT) or magnetic resonance imaging (MRI) before surgery. In other cases, a judgment decision of the operation was made by a surgeon.

Operative technique

All operations were carried out by experienced shoulder surgeons. There were 53 patients in the Bankart repair group (33 males). The patient was placed in the lateral decubitus position, and the arm was abducted approximately 45° with longitudinal traction. When performing Bankart repair, the cartilage of the anterior border of the scapula was first cleaned and the anterior and posterior capsule sacral lip complex was freshened. Then, the damaged anterior and inferior joint capsule sacral lip complex was completely released. The suture anchor (Lupine BR Anchor, DePuy Mitek, Raynham, MA, the USA) was evenly placed on the cartilage surface of the glenoid for repair, and the suture was introduced into the labrum by a suturing device and knotted.

There were 52 patients in the Latarjet group (34 males). The shoulder joint was in the abduction and external rotation, so that the coracoacromial ligament was revealed. The coracoacromial ligament was divided 1 cm lateral to the coracoid, and the coracoid was osteotomized at its base. Then, two drill holes were pre-drilled through the coracoid. The anteroinferior aspect of the labrum was excised. The coracoid bone was fixed to the glenoid rim through the subscapularis tendon with malleolar screws. The stump of the coracoacromial ligament was sutured to the most medial aspect of the joint capsule (Figure 1).

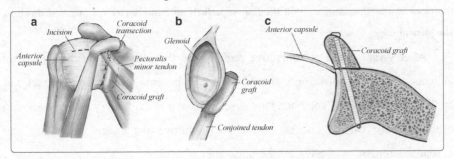

Figure 1   a. An inverted L-shaped opening (dotted line) is made in the anterior approach to form the capsule flap from the glenoid neck. Pectoralis minor (dotted line) is detached from the coracoid before the coracoid osteotomy is carried out. b. Coracoid graft is fixed to glenoid rim with 2 malleolar screws. If the curve is not fit, the graft can be re-sharpened. c. Put the graft onto glenoid rim as an extension of the articular platform

There were 45 patients in the capsular shift group (31 males). For capsular shift, the incision started several centimeters below the tip of the condyle and proceeded to the inferior border of the pectoralis major muscle. The subscapularis tendon was incised 1 cm medial to its insertion on the lesser tuberosity, and the muscular position of the subscapularis was also separated from the capsule. The capsular flaps were repaired. When the capsule had been sufficiently mobilized, the capsule was anchored medially to the glenoid with suture anchors (Mitek G2

Anchor, Raynham, MA, the USA). The capsule was split in "T" or "L" fashion, then the inferior flap was pulled superiorly, and was sutured to the lateral capsular remnant. The capsular cleft between the superior and middle glenohumeral ligaments was closed and reinforced the capsule anteriorly (Figure 2).

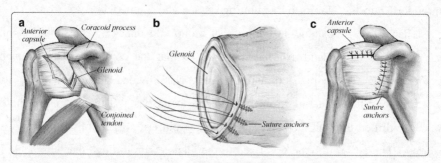

Figure 2   a. The capsule is incised based on inverted "L" shape to expose glenoid rim adequately. b. Three to four suture anchors are positioned medially from 3 o'clock to 6 o'clock to the direction. c. Pull the flap superiorly to make incise capsule tied down to the glenoid edge

After surgery, the postoperative regime was the same for the three groups. Patients were immobilized in a shoulder brace in internal rotation for 6 weeks and applied ice around the shoulder joint within 3 days after surgery. Active motion exercises were carried out as tolerated to improve the range of motion and muscular strength by a physical therapist after 6 weeks.

Outcome measures

All patients were assessed by one observer, independent of the operating surgeons, with a questionnaire that included stability, satisfaction, subjective shoulder value (SSV), subjective shoulder value for sport practice (SSV Sport), the American Shoulder and Elbow Joint Surgery Association shoulder joint score (ASES), Rowe score, University of California at Los Angeles scoring system (UCLA score), and external rotation (ER). ER was measured with the elbow at 90° of abduction using a goniometer. Hyperlaxity was defined as the small resistance and large rotation angle of ER (ER > 85°). We ranked SSV and SSV Sport between 0% and 100% to assess activities of daily living. 150 patients were followed up at a minimum of 36 months. The average follow-up was

57.6 months (range 36 – 72).

Statistical methods

Statistical analysis was analyzed by SPSS. The chi-square test was used to assess differences between categorical data. Data were described as mean ± standard deviation. The significance level was set at a P value of less than 0.05.

Results

Functional results

The Rowe score in the arthroscopic Bankart repair group was higher than the other two groups with statistical significance ($P < 0.05$). Latarjet was lower in the poor Rowe level ($P < 0.05$). Compared to joint motion, external rotations on the affected side were 81.3 ± 3.1°, 79.8 ± 2.5°, and 78.5 ± 3.5° with no statistical significance ($P > 0.05$). No significant association was found between other outcome measures (Table 2).

Table 2　Functional results

Variable	Bankart ($n = 53$)	Latarjet ($n = 52$)	Capsular shift ($n = 45$)
ASES (mean ± SD)	92.12 ± 1.83	91.54 ± 2.38	92.41 ± 1.81
UCLA score (mean ± SD)	29.40 ± 1.12	31.83 ± 1.35	31.13 ± 1.62
Hyperlaxity (ER > 85°) (%)	41 (77.4%)	38 (73.1%)	33 (73.3%)
Rowe score(mean ± SD)	92.36 ± 1.5]	96.23 ± 2.10*	93.22 ± 2.31
Rowe level			
Excellent (90 – 100)(%)	27 (50.9%)	28 (53.8%)	24 (53.3%)
Good (75 – 89)(%)	18 (34.0%)	20 (38.5%)	15 (33.3%)
Fair (40 – 74)(%)	3 (5.7%)	2 (3.8%)	3 (6.7%)
Poor (0 – 39)(%)	5 (9.4%)	2 (3.8%)*	3 (6.7%)

ASES American Shoulder and Elbow Joint Surgery Association shoulder joint score; *ER* external rotation. *$P < 0.05$.

Subjective results

Interestingly, there were no significant differences in satisfaction among these groups ($P > 0.05$). However, the analysis showed better subjective results after Latarjet with respect to SSV Sport. The SSV Sport in the Latarjet group was superior to the Bankart group. By comparison, the capsular shift group had the lowest value ($P < 0.05$). Similar to the previous result, the capsular shift seemed to score the worst values in SSV ($P < 0.05$), as shown in Table 3.

Table 3 Subjective results

Variable	Bankart ($n = 53$)	Latarjet ($n = 52$)	Capsular shift ($n = 45$)
Very satisfied + satisfied (%)	47 (88.7%)	48 (92.3%)	37 (82.2%)
SSV (%)	50 (10% – 100%)	50 (30% – 100%)	39 (10% – 100%) [*]
SSV Sport (%)	41 (0% – 100%) [*]	44 (0% – 100%) [*]	33 (0% – 100%) [*]

SSV: subjective shoulder value. SSV sport: subjective shoulder value for sport practice. [*] $P < 0.05$.

Complications

Five patients had a temporary postoperative complication. In the arthroscopic Bankart repair group, there were one postoperative hematoma along the arm and one transient musculocutaneous nerve palsy. In the open Latarjet group, there were two postoperative hematomas along the axillary fold and arm. In the capsular shift group, there was just one case who had a transient musculocutaneous nerve palsy. All postoperative hematomas were resorbed spontaneously after 6 weeks, and all cases who had a transient musculocutaneous nerve palsy recovered spontaneously after 6 months. Of course, none of them had any residual sequelae.

Recurrence

One patient in the arthroscopic Bankart group (1.9%) and one in the capsular shift group (2.2%) had a postoperative recurrence. The former occurred after 2 years when the patient played basketball, and the latter was caused by a fall after 17 months. The Latarjet group had no recurrence.

Discussion

With the development of arthroscopy, arthroscopic Bankart repair has already been widely used to treat recurrent anterior shoulder instability, which took away open surgery as the gold standard. To our knowledge, existing reports hold different attitudes, causing a fair amount of confusion, so that surgeons relied more on their experience due to the lack of guidelines.

Interestingly, our study found that patients undergoing Latarjet procedures could achieve significantly better stability, subjective perception for sport practice, and lower recurrence compared with the other two. This study also demonstrated that Bankart repair had no advantages in terms of external rotation and other outcome measure scores comparing open surgical procedures. In addition, the operation of Bankart repair did not decrease the number of complications from our study. However, considering that our study was still limited by sample size, we cannot tell whether differences of complications requiring reoperation remained statistically significant.

Several prior reports also revealed that open Latarjet surgery appeared with better results, while opposite results were reported by others. In our study, we used the Rowe score to assess postoperative stability, which contained stability, motion, and function. In terms of postoperative stability, Latarjet procedures may be more advisable. We considered that the triple effect of anterior glenoid augmentation, the capsular repair, and the sling effect of the conjoined tendon may strengthen the efficacy, especially in significant structural bone deficits. But Latarjet procedures were not without defects. Matthes et al. have found the loss of elevation or internal and external rotation after the Latarjet procedure. Facts proved that it coincided with our clinical practice despite a shortage of comparative researches. By contrast, Petrera et al. reported that patients undergoing modern arthroscopic Bankart repair showed better return to sport compared with open technique. Uehara et al. also reported a similar result about Bankart repair and return to previous activity level.

Besides, it was also controversial that the loss of range of motion (ROM) after arthroscopic Bankart repair was minor to that after open capsular repair. Some meta-analysis studies reported that Bankart repair can provide better recovery of ER at 90° abduction. However, other studies indicated no significant difference in loss of ROM. We compared the number of perioperative hyperlaxity (ER > 85°), and then, there was no difference in ER. However, we did not measure specific changes of angle, resulting in a certain error due to their uncertainty.

In the view of many surgeons, there was a lower risk of complications for Bankart repair compared with open surgery. However, our study did not support this viewpoint. The incidence of complications of Bankart repair was higher than the others. Fortunately, there were two postoperative hematomas along the axillary fold and arm without loosening of fixation or small coracoid in the Latarjet group. Some reports revealed that the majority of complications of Latarjet procedure were related to a technical error and implant failure. In such cases, some studies suggested choosing another surgical to avoid this complication due to lack of appropriate screwing fixation. According to our experience, a rigorous selection of patients who had small coracoid was the key to the success of Latarjet procedure. For Bankart repair, the current large amount of researches argued that Bankart repair had fewer associated complications, including infection, nerve palsy, and internal rotation contractures. This view was not supported in our study.

With respect to recurrence, our recurrence rate was 1.9% in the arthroscopic Bankart group, 0% in the Latarjet group, and 2.2% in the capsular shift group. We were delighted with this outcome in comparison with the classical arthroscopic Bankart surgery varying from 8% to 64%. Of these patients, one undergoing Bankart repair had re-dislocation after 2 years when playing basketball and one undergoing capsular shift occurred by a fall after 17 months. It indicated the potential factors of dislocation still existed after operation. For capsular shift, despite the good results from the beginning, a long-term effect (maybe over 5 years) was still uncertain according to the paper by Hovelius et al. Burkhart and De Beer reported that glenoid bone loss greater than 25% led to a high risk of recurrence for arthroscopic Bankart repair, whereas recurrence was only 4% without bone loss. Hence, we recommended Latarjet procedure to treat redislocation patients who had a higher request for activities and the absence of bone loss.

Overall, all three treatments proved to be effective in improving shoulder functional status and reducing symptoms. All of them had a satisfying result, and 118 cases returned to sports at the preinjury level at the final follow-up. The number of patients with a permanent incapacity for work was negligible in three groups. We can see the same results from the paper by Mohtadi et al. However, it was clear from this study that Bankart repair, Latarjet procedures, and capsular shift still had a lot of room to develop in treatment concept and technique of anterior shoulder instability. Take Latarjet technique as an example, it often presented an obvious challenge for junior doctors. To some extent, we can diminish these confounding factors by improving technique and training. Even so, there was still a certain rate of failure for an experienced surgeon because we cannot predict the evolution of the variable graft healing when undergoing Latarjet procedure. One interesting thing we found was that most Chinese patients, especially older patients, were more willing to use complimentary care modalities or Bankart repair due to rapid recovery. Actually, according to years of experience, capsular shift can be a good alternative if facing anteroinferior or multidirectional type of shoulder, but not including severe bone defect. As for the limitation of the thesis, further study was still demanded in this field.

By combining the clinical practice, some suggestions can be offered here to determine which patient is best suited to each surgical. Arthroscopic Bankart repair has the advantages of mini-invasion and rapid recovery. Capsular shift offers the advantage of stabilizing multidirectional type of shoulder. Latarjet can provide greater stability with low recurrence. At the same time, open Latarjet better suits young active patients, especially those with contact sports.

Conclusions

The results revealed that all treatments were effective in improving shoulder functional status and reducing symptoms.

However, open Latarjet procedure is more reliable in terms of shoulder stability and subjective perception than the others. In clinical practice, we still need to choose the optimal operative management on each specific matter, and here, we sum up some experience as reference: ① Arthroscopic Bankart repair has the advantages of mini-invasion and rapid recovery. ② Capsular shift has the advantages of stabilizing anteroinferior or multidirectional type of shoulder. ③ Latarjet was more effective in reducing recurrence with higher stability and has better subjective perception.

JOSR. 2019; 14(1):326

DOI: 10.1186/s13018 - 019 - 1340 - 5

词汇

instability	n. 不稳定(性);基础薄弱;不安定
recurrence	n. 复发;循环;重现
avulsion	n. 扯开,撕裂;扯离的部分
capsule	n. 胶囊;太空舱;小容器
questionnaire	n. 问卷;调查表
tendon	n. [解剖]腱
rigorous	adj. 严格的,严厉的;严密的;严酷的
arthroscopic	adj. 关节镜的
hyperlaxity	n. 过度松弛
glenohumeral	adj. 盂肱的

译文

三种术式治疗复发性肩关节前脱位的疗效比较:
关节镜下 Bankart 损伤修复术、Latarjet 手术、关节囊紧缩移位术

摘要

背景 复发性肩关节前脱位的最佳手术治疗方式仍存在争议。我们对传统开放手术和现代的关节镜技术的优势和选择知之甚少。我们假设,无论采用何种手术技术,所有患者的疗效都是相似的。

方法 我们对 2010 年 9 月至 2013 年 12 月的 168 例复发性肩关节前脱位患者进行了回顾性病例队列分析。所有病例(年龄为 18—50 岁,平均年龄为 30.8 岁)均接受了关节镜下 Bankart 损伤修复术(男 33 例,女 20 例)、切开 Latarjet 手术(男 34 例,女 18 例)、关节囊紧缩移位术(男 31 例,女 14 例)。随访时间为 60 ~ 72 个月,平均为 67.6 个月。肩关节不稳定严重程度指数(ISIS)评分均大于 3 分,平均为 6.4 分。

结果 所有治疗方法均能有效改善肩关节的功能状态、减轻症状,而切开 Latarjet 手术组在主观感受方面具有优势。关节镜下 Bankart 损伤修复术组、切开 Latarjet 手术组和关节囊紧缩移位术组的 Rowe 评分分别为 92.3±1.5 分、96.2±2.1 分和 93.2±2.3 分,差异有统计学意义。其他功能结果无显著差异。

但在主观结果［主观肩关节估值(SSV)和主观肩关节运动估值(SSV Sport)］方面,Latarjet手术组明显优于其他两组($P<0.05$)。关节镜下Bankart损伤修复术组和关节囊紧缩移位术组分别有2例复发,而切开Latarjet手术组无复发病例。

结论 关节镜下Bankart损伤修复术具有创伤小、恢复快等优点。关节囊紧缩移位术可以提供下方或多向型的稳定,特别是对于合并微小骨缺损的病例。Latarjet手术在减少复发方面效果更好,术后具有更高的稳定性。

证据水平 治疗Ⅲ级

关键词 肩关节 脱位 Bankart损伤修复术 Latarjet手术 关节囊紧缩移位术

前言

复发性肩关节前脱位是肩胛盂前缘撕脱及前下方关节囊不可逆拉伸所致,被称为"Bankart损伤"。据报道,其发病率高达60%,并处于上升趋势。合并严重的关节盂和关节囊缺损复发性肩关节前脱位的最佳手术治疗方式仍然具有挑战性。这是一种致残性的疾病,我们通常采用关节镜下Bankart损伤修复术、切开Latarjet手术及关节囊紧缩移位术来治疗。

随着关节镜技术的发展,Bankart损伤修复术已成为目前治疗复发性肩关节前脱位的首选方法,近90%的外科医生采用此种术式。多项研究表明,与其他方法相比,Bankart损伤修复术可以保证肩关节有较强的稳定性,并且术后复发较少。然而,也有反对者指出,目前的研究中存在着潜在干扰因素,这些因素可能与预后差异有关,包括性别、年龄、关节囊过度松弛、脱位史、运动水平、肩胛骨肱骨端的病变等。此外,这些技术的复发性在文献中的一致性也不高。他们认为手术的侧重点应该是解剖修复,这恰恰是Bankart损伤修复术无法做到的。如今,肱盂关节骨缺损和关节囊缺损在肩关节前脱位中仍然普遍存在。它被称为Broca-Perthes-Bankart(关节囊松弛和盂肱韧带撕脱复合损伤)。Latarjet手术已被证明是安全可靠的,它可以弥补Bankart损伤修复术的不足,并且术后的复发率更低。此外,关节囊紧缩移位术在美国被广泛使用,因为它同样可以解决Bankart损伤及关节囊松弛的问题。这三种术式现已成为手术治疗复发性肩关节前脱位的主流术式。然而,根据现有的研究结果,我们对传统开放手术和现代关节镜技术的优缺点还没有足够的了解。目前仍没有确切的术式选择建议,因此术式的选择往往取决于医生的习惯和偏好。

对于外科医生来说,掌握Bankart损伤修复术和开放手术的相关知识是非常重要的,这可以提供准确的术前风险和术后疗效评估。在这项研究中,我们采用更大的样本量和更长的随访时间(至少 36 个月)评估这三种治疗方法。这项研究的目的是评估这些手术的功能和主观结果,并确定哪种手术更满足需要。

材料与方法

患者

2010 年 9 月至 2013 年 12 月,我们进行了一项回顾性研究,以分析我们医院复发性肩关节前脱位患者的疗效。这项研究计划得到了当地伦理委员会的批准,并获得了同意。

患者均以复发性肩关节前脱位为主要诊断结果,他们在轻微外力下即发生肩关节脱位,病程至少一年。同时,我们对 18—50 岁年龄组的受试者进行随机抽样。其他纳入标准:肩关节不稳定严重程度指数评分(ISIS)得分至少为 3 分;有较高的运动需求(尤其是过肩运动)。排除标准:肩关节骨性关节炎(关节间隙有明显改变);多向的复发性肩关节半脱位或脱位;首次脱位;严重癫痫;骨骺尚未闭合;严重的肩关节盂骨缺损(正位 X 线片上的关节盂轮廓丧失);活动期感染性疾病;严重内科疾病。最终,我们筛选出符合上述纳入、排除标准的 102 例患者。其中 11 名患者的数据不完整,其余 91 名患者(平均年龄为 30.8 岁,范围在 18—50 岁,右肩 62 例,ISIS 平均分为 6.4 分)的随访时间为至少 36 个月。根据不同的术式(Bankart 损伤修复术、Latarjet 手术和关节囊紧缩移位术),患者被分为三组。人口学数据和术前功能评分在三组之间并无统计学差异(表 1)。

表 1　人口学数据和术前特征

变量	Bankart 损伤修复术 ($n = 53$)	Latarjet 手术 ($n = 52$)	关节囊紧缩移位术 ($n = 45$)
年龄(岁,平均数 ± 标准差)	29.81 ± 4.31	31.23 ± 6.12	30.75 ± 3.85
男性/女性	33/20	34/18	31/14
优势侧	37	32	31
病程(月,平均数 ± 标准差)	14.25 ± 5.10	13.80 ± 3.13	13.42 ± 3.72
对抗性运动(%)	26(49.1%)	20(38.5%)	24(53.3%)
过度松弛(ER > 85°)(%)	27(51.0%)	24(46.2%)	21(46.7%)
Rowe 评分(平均数 ± 标准差)	48.74 ± 12.08	42.23 ± 14.20	50.87 ± 9.61
ISIS(平均数 ± 标准差)	6.16 ± 2.81	7.01 ± 3.02	6.50 ± 2.56

ER:外旋角度;ISIS:不稳定严重程度指数。对抗性运动:球类、投掷类、体操类等。$P < 0.05$ 被认为具有统计学意义。

根据术前常规 CT 或 MRI 检查，如果关节盂前缘丢失大于关节盂的最大前后径的 50% 以上，则考虑采用 Latarjet 手术。在其他情况下，术式的选择取决于外科医生自身。

手术技术

　　所有手术均由经验丰富的肩关节外科医生完成。Bankart 损伤修复术组有 53 例患者（男性 33 例）。患者取侧卧位，活动肩关节，患侧手臂 45°纵向牵引。在实施 Bankart 损伤修复术时，首先清理肩胛盂前缘的损伤软骨组织，将其前下方关节囊盂唇复合体新鲜化，然后松解损伤的前下方关节囊盂唇复合体。之后将缝合锚钉（美国马萨诸塞州雷纳姆的 DePuy Mitek 公司的 Lupine BR 型锚钉）均匀打入肩胛盂软骨表面进行修复，通过缝合器将缝线引入盂唇内并进行打结固定。

　　Latarjet 手术组有 52 例患者（男性 34 例）。术中肩关节外展外旋，显露喙肩韧带。喙肩韧带在喙突外 1 厘米处断开，于喙突基底部截骨。然后，在喙突上预先钻取两个钻孔，修整肩胛盂前下部。喙突通过肩胛下肌腱被踝关节螺钉固定在关节缘。喙肩韧带的残端被缝合在关节囊的最内侧（图 1）。

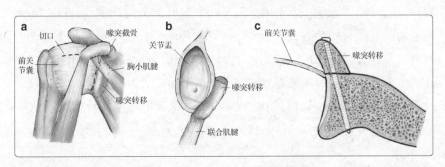

　　图 1　a. 前入路形成倒"L"形开口（虚线），形成囊膜瓣。在进行喙突截骨前，先将胸小肌（虚线）从喙突分离。b. 喙突骨块被 2 枚踝关节螺钉固定于关节缘。如果曲线不合适，可以打磨骨块。c. 将骨块置于关节缘，作为关节平台的延伸

　　关节囊紧缩移位术组有 45 例患者（男性 31 例）。手术切口从肩峰以下数厘米开始，一直到胸大肌下缘。肩胛下肌腱在小结节止点内侧 1 厘米处被切开，分离肩胛下肌与关节囊。修复肩关节囊瓣。关节囊被分离后，用缝合锚钉（美国马萨诸塞州雷纳姆的 Mitek G2 锚钉）将关节囊向内侧固定在肩胛盂上。"T"或"L"形切开关节囊，向上牵拉囊瓣，将其缝合于外侧关节囊残端。闭合盂肱上、中韧带之间的关节囊切口，对前方关节囊进行加强缝合（图 2）。

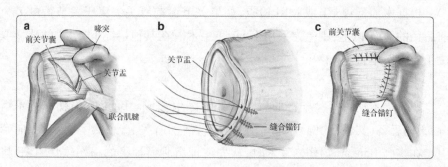

图 2 **a.** 关节囊以倒"L"形切开,充分暴露肩胛盂边缘。**b.** 将三个到四个缝合锚钉置于内侧,从 3 点钟方向到 6 点钟方向。**c.** 向上拉动囊瓣,将切开的囊膜与肩胛盂边缘缝合在一起

三组患者的术后康复计划相同。术后 3 天内患肩冰敷,肩关节支具内旋位置固定肩关节 6 周。6 周后渐进性进行外旋、外展等主动活动(由专业的理疗师进行康复指导),从而扩大术后肩关节的运动范围及恢复上肢肌力。

主要指标

所有患者均由一名与手术医生无关联的观察者进行评估,问卷内容包括稳定性、满意度、主观肩关节估值(SSV)、主观肩关节运动估值(SSV Sport)、美国肩肘关节外科协会肩关节评分(ASES)、Rowe 评分、美国加州大学洛杉矶分校肩关节评分系统(UCLA 评分)及肩关节外旋角度(ER)。ER 是曲肘 90°时用测角器测量的。过度松弛被定义为"小阻力和大外旋展角"(ER > 85°)。SSV 估值和 SSV Sport 估值采用 0% ~ 100% 来评估患者的日常活动情况。150 例患者至少被随访了 36 个月。随访时间为 36 ~ 72 个月,平均时间为57.6 个月。

统计学分析

本次研究采用 SPSS 统计软件进行分析。卡方检验用于评估分类数据之间的差异,数据描述为平均值 ± 标准偏差,$P < 0.05$ 被认为差异具有统计学意义。

结果

功能活动评价

关节镜下 Bankart 损伤修复术组的 Rowe 评分高于其他两组,差异有统计学意义($P < 0.05$)。Latarjet 手术组的 Rowe 评分较低($P < 0.05$)。比较关节活动,患侧关节外旋角度分别为 81.3° ±3.1°、79.8° ±2.5°、78.5° ±3.5°,差异

无统计学意义（$P > 0.05$）。我们没有发现其他结果指标之间存在显著的相关性（表2）。

表2 功能结果

变量	Bankart 损伤修复术 （$n = 53$）	Latarjet 手术 （$n = 52$）	关节囊紧缩移位术 （$n = 45$）
ASES 评分（平均值±标准方差）	92.12 ± 1.83	91.54 ± 2.38	92.41 ± 1.81
UCLA 评分（平均值±标准方差）	29.40 ± 1.12	31.83 ± 1.35	31.13 ± 1.62
过度松弛（ER > 85°）（%）	41（77.4%）	38（73.1%）	33（73.3%）
Rowe 评分（平均值±标准方差）	92.36 ± 1.51	96.23 ± 2.10 *	93.22 ± 2.31
Rowe 水平（平均值±标准方差）			
极好（90—100）（%）	27（50.9%）	28（53.8%）	24（53.3%）
好（75—89）（%）	18（34.0%）	20（38.5%）	15（33.3%）
不好（40—74）（%）	3（5.7%）	2（3.8%）	3（6.7%）
差（0—39）（%）	5（9.4%）	2（3.8%）*	3（6.7%）

ASES：美国肩肘关节外科协会肩关节评分；ER：外旋角度。*$P < 0.05$。

主观感受评价

三组患者术后的满意度差异并没有统计学意义（$P > 0.05$）。然而，分析表明 Latarjet 手术组的主观感受评价更好，且主观肩关节运动估值（SSV Sport）高于 Bankart 损伤修复术组，在主观肩关节运动估值（SSV Sport）方面，关节囊紧缩移位术组主观肩关节运动估值（SSV Sport）最低，且差异具有统计学意义（$P < 0.05$）。关节囊紧缩移位术组在主观肩关节估值（SSV）的评价中同样也最差，差异具有统计学意义（$P < 0.05$）（表3）。

表3 主观结果

变量	Bankart 损伤修复术 （$n = 53$）	Latarjet 手术 （$n = 52$）	关节囊紧缩移位术 （$n = 45$）
非常满意 + 满意（%）	47（88.7%）	48（92.3%）	37（82.2%）
SSV 估值（%）	50（10%～100%）	50（30%～100%）	39（10%～100%）*
SSV Sport 估值（%）	41（0%～100%）*	44（0%～100%）*	33（0%～100%）*

SSV：主观肩关节估值；SSV Sport：主观肩关节运动估值。*$P < 0.05$。

术后并发症

术后出现一过性并发症5例。关节镜下 Bankart 损伤修复术组出现1例术后上臂血肿及1例短暂性肌皮神经麻痹。Latarjet 手术组有2例术后腋窝及上臂的血肿。关节囊紧缩移位术组中出现 1 例短暂性肌皮神经麻痹。术后 6 周,血肿均被吸收;短暂性肌皮神经麻痹 6 个月后也全部恢复正常。患者均无其他后遗症。

脱位复发

关节镜下 Bankart 损伤修复术组中有 1 例(1.9%)术后肩关节脱位复发,关节囊紧缩移位术组中也有 1 例(2.2%)术后复发。前者是在术后 2 年打篮球时发生的,后者是术后 17 个月时不慎跌倒所致。而 Latarjet 手术组暂时未发现术后脱位复发病例。

讨论

随着关节镜技术的迅猛发展,关节镜下 Bankart 损伤修复术已被广泛应用于复发性肩关节前脱位的手术治疗,不再以切开手术为治疗的黄金标准。现有的文献对此持有不同的观点,这在临床中给我们造成相当多的困惑。由于缺乏权威指南,骨科医生在临床中更多地依赖自身经验进行术式选择。

我们发现,与其他两组患者相比,接受 Latarjet 手术的患者能够获得更高的肩关节稳定性,术后运动锻炼的主观感受也明显更好,并且术后更不容易出现脱位复发。这项研究还表明,与其他术式相比,关节镜下 Bankart 损伤修复术在肩关节外旋角度和其他结果评分方面并没有明显优势。此外,关节镜下 Bankart 损伤修复术也并没有减少术后并发症。然而,考虑我们的研究仍然受到了样本量的限制,我们并不能判断三种术式出现需要二次手术的并发症的组间差异是否具有统计学意义。

之前的一些文献显示,Latarjet 手术的疗效更好,但也有一部分文献的结果正好相反。在本次研究中,我们用 Rowe 评分来评估肩关节术后的稳定性,包括肩关节稳定性、运动情况及功能恢复情况。在术后稳定性方面,Latarjet 手术更为可取。因此,我们认为前肩胛盂的延伸、肩关节囊的修复和联合肌腱的牵拉这三重效应可以增强手术的疗效,尤其是在显著的结构性骨缺损方面。但是,Latarjet 手术也并不是没有缺陷。Matthes 等人发现在进行 Latarjet 手术后,患者可能会出现患肩上举或内外旋活动的受限。尽管这个结论缺乏数据支持,但在临床上是存在的。而 Petrera 等人称,接受关节镜下 Bankart 损伤修复术的患者比接受开放手术的患者术后更能达到运动恢复的目的。对于关节镜下 Bankart 损伤修复术及术后运动水平的恢复情况,Uehara 等人的研究也得到类似的结果。

此外,与关节囊紧缩移位术相比,关节镜下 Bankart 损伤修复术的术后肩关节活动度(ROM)的损失较少,这一点也存在争议。有一些元分析研究指出,关节镜下 Bankart 损伤修复术能够更好地恢复患肩 90°外展时的外旋角度。然而,其他研究却表明,在肩关节活动度的损失程度方面,两者并没有显著差异。比较两组患者围术期肩关节过度松弛的次数(ER > 85°),并无太大组间差异。但是,我们并没有比较其他特定角度时的变化,这可能造成一定的误差。

根据许多外科医生的观点,与开放手术相比,关节镜下 Bankart 损伤修复术发生术后并发症的风险更低。然而,这一观点在本次研究中没有得到支持。本次研究中,关节镜下 Bankart 损伤修复术组的术后并发症的发生率比其他两组高。而 Latarjet 手术组术后虽然出现 2 例腋窝或上臂的血肿,但并没有出现内固定或喙突骨块松动的情况。一些研究表明,大多数 Latarjet 手术的术后并发症的发生与手术失误及植入物固定失败有关。在这种情况下,一些研究建议,如果缺乏合适的固定螺丝,可采用别的术式来避免这种并发症。根据我们的经验,喙突截骨患者的严格选择是 Latarjet 手术成功的关键。对于 Bankart 损伤修复术,当前大量研究提出,Bankart 损伤修复术的相关术后并发症更少,包括感染、神经麻痹和内旋挛缩。这一观点并没有得到本研究的支持。

在术后脱位复发方面,关节镜下 Bankart 损伤修复术组的复发率为 1.9%,Latarjet 手术组为 0%,关节囊紧缩移位术组为 2.2%。与传统的关节镜下 Bankart 损伤手术的 8%～64% 的复发率相比,我们对本研究的结果非常满意。一例接受关节镜下 Bankart 损伤修复术治疗的患者在术后 2 年进行篮球运动时发生肩关节再次脱位,另一例再次脱位是关节囊紧缩移位术后 17 个月时跌倒所致。这提醒我们术后脱位的潜在因素仍然存在。对于关节囊紧缩移位术,尽管术后的恢复效果良好,但根据 Hovelius 等人的研究,其长期疗效(或许 5 年以上)仍不确定。Burkhart 和 De Beer 称,接受关节镜下 Bankart 损伤修复术治疗的患者中,超过 25% 的肩关节盂骨缺损是导致肩关节脱位复发的高危因素,而在没有骨缺损的情况下,术后脱位复发率仅为 4%。因此,对于术后运动要求高及存在骨缺损的脱位患者,我们建议采用 Latarjet 手术治疗。

总的来说,这三种术式在改善肩关节功能及减轻症状方面都被证明是有效的。患者均获得了满意的效果,118 例患者在最后一次随访中恢复到了伤前运动水平。三组患者中,没有永久丧失工作能力的患者。我们可以从 Mohtadi

等人的文献中看到同样的结果。然而,这项研究表明,关节镜下 Bankart 损伤修复术、Latarjet 手术及关节囊紧缩移位术在复发性肩关节前脱位的治疗观念及技术方面仍有很大的发展空间。以 Latarjet 手术为例,它对于经验不足的年轻医生来说是很大的挑战。在一定程度上,我们可以通过手术技术改进及大量的训练来减少这些困难。即便如此,由于移植骨块愈合的不确定性,Latarjet 手术对于经验丰富的外科医生来说仍存在一定的失败率。有趣的是,大多数中国患者,特别是老年患者,由于康复速度快,更愿意采用保守治疗或接受 Bankart 损伤修复术治疗。事实上,根据我们多年的工作经验,对于前下或多向型,但不包括严重骨缺损的肩关节脱位,关节囊紧缩移位术是很好的选择。由于研究的局限性,这方面还有待进一步研究。

通过结合临床,我们在这里可以提供一些建议,以确定患者最适合哪一种手术:关节镜下 Bankart 损伤修复术具有创伤小、恢复快的优点;关节囊紧缩移位术能够提供多向的稳定性;Latarjet 手术拥有较低的术后复发率及更高的肩关节稳定性。我们建议活动较多的年轻患者接受 Latarjet 手术,尤其是有进行身体接触运动需求的患者。

结论

所有治疗方法均能有效改善肩关节功能,减轻症状。

然而,Latarjet 手术在肩关节稳定性和患者主观感受方面比其他两种术式更为可靠。在临床上,我们仍须针对具体情况选择最佳的手术方式,在此总结一些经验以供参考:① 关节镜下 Bankart 损伤修复术具有微创、恢复快的优点。② 关节囊紧缩移位术具有前下或多向型稳定的优点。③ Latarjet 手术能够保证更高的肩关节稳定性,术后脱位复发率更低,患者的主观感受也更好。

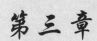

第三章

标题的拟定与作者署名

3.1　标题的拟定

标题(title)是吸引读者去浏览摘要和阅读文章的第一步,给读者提供论文的最核心信息,应起到画龙点睛的作用。标题是整篇论文被阅读次数最多的部分,也有可能是唯一被阅读的部分。标题可以视为作者为整篇论文制作的"面具",要有代表性和吸引力,以便读者可以据此快速判断论文的价值及与自己研究的相关性,从而决定是否继续阅读论文。由此可见,标题的拟定至关重要。

不同的英文期刊对标题的格式要求不同,一般分为两种:一种是期刊第一个单词的首字母大写,其余都小写;另一种是每个实词的首字母均大写,虚词小写。部分期刊要求包含四个字母以上的虚词也要大写(第一个单词的首字母须大写,不管是实词还是虚词)。专有名词的首字母和缩略词都要大写。具体格式要根据不同期刊的要求做出调整。

标题看似简单,但一不注意就容易出现与论文具体内容产生偏差的问题。论文的标题应该精确(accuracy)、简练(brevity)和严谨(strictness),既可以用最简洁的语言准确描述、高度概括论文的内容和主题,又可以吸引读者。需要注意的是,精确是最重要的。

(1)精确

标题一定要精确,用词要有专业性,符合文章的具体内容,不要用太宽泛的词汇描述,这样标题才能更加明确并且具有较强的信息性,从而准确反映研究和论文的主要内容。可以使用研究的重要术语,最好能够与关键词形成互补,这样能够为读者提供关于这篇论文的更多信息。拟定标题时可以围绕以下三个要点进行:核心问题,即研究想解决的难题;主要结果,即研究取得的最有价值的结果;主要结论,即由研究结果得出的核心结论。

(2)简练

标题要简洁明了,用尽量少的文字概括尽量多的内容。很多英文期刊对标题的字数是有严格限制的,最好不要超过 12 个英文实词,但也不能为追求简短而过于忽视内容的表述,这样可能会使读者产生错误的理解,给读者造成阅读障碍。我们可以将核心词置于标题,从而清晰地表述出论文的特色与具体内容。英文标题多由名词性短语构成,少数也可以是一个完整的语句,但都必须言简意赅,用最少的词把核心内容说清楚。当标题是个完整的句子时,结尾一般不用加句号。在汉语标题中,我们常常使用"研究""关于""问题""体会""经验""探讨"等没有实质性内容的词汇,而我们在英文论文标题中往往对此类词汇不予采用。

(3)严谨

医学是一门严谨的科学,论文标题也应尽可能严谨。通常标题中应尽量少出现缩写和首字母缩略词,以免妨碍读者的快速阅读,要做到使读者不必了解论文的其他部分内容便能理解标题包含的所有信息。不能单单为了追求标题的简练而使其表意不明。标题常常由名词性短语构成,所以词序及修饰关系就至关重要,如果使用修饰关系不当,往往会使读者产生理解偏差。我们有时还可以使用副标题来对主标题进行进一步说明,副标题要用冒号或破折号与主标题分开。但一般情况下,为了使标题简练,也为了方便文献的检索,尽量不要使用副标题。

示 例

以下为英文论文标题拟定的几种常用类型及示例。

(1)描述对研究对象的比较与研究对象的相关性

①3D 打印导航辅助与徒手应用寰枢椎椎弓根螺钉治疗 II 型齿状突骨折的对比研究

Comparative study of 3D printed navigation template-assisted atlantoaxial pedicle screws versus free-hand screws for type II odontoid fractures

② 两种髋关节重建技术的生物力学比较：自体髂胫束移植与同种异体跟腱移植

A Biomechanical Comparison of 2 Hip Capsular Reconstruction Techniques：Iliotibial Band Autograft Versus Achilles Tendon Allograft

③ 女性骨关节炎患者口服双膦酸盐与骨髓病变体积的关系

The relation of oral bisphosphonates to bone marrow lesion volume among women with osteoarthritis

④ 软骨钙化与骨性关节炎：病理联系？

Cartilage calcification and osteoarthritis：a pathological association？

⑤ 保留梨状肌的微创手术与标准后路全髋关节置换术：10 年随访的随机对照试验

Piriformis-Sparing Minimally Invasive Versus the Standard Posterior Approach for Total Hip Arthroplasty：A 10-Year Follow-Up of a Randomized Control Trial

⑥ 降雨与关节痛或背痛的关系：回顾性分析

Association between rainfall and diagnoses of joint or back pain：retrospective claims analysis

⑦ 内科、外科医生的高尔夫球习惯：观察性队列研究

Golf habits among physicians and surgeons：observational cohort study

⑧ 男、女外科医生治疗的术后疗效比较：配对队列研究

Comparison of postoperative outcomes among patients treated by male and female surgeons：a population based matched cohort study

（2）描述研究对象的效果、影响、临床价值等

① 辛伐他汀在大鼠骨质疏松模型和股骨缺损模型中的成骨作用

Osteogenic effects in a rat osteoporosis model and femur defect model by simvastatin microcrystals

② 对运动员进行籽骨切除术的功能效果

Functional Outcome of Sesamoid Excision in Athletes

③ 刮除术对骨巨细胞瘤局部控制的影响

The impact of curettage technique on local control in giant cell tumour of bone

④ 关节镜下肩胛上神经减压术治疗肩胛上神经病的临床疗效

Clinical Outcomes of Arthroscopic Suprascapular Nerve Decompression for Suprascapular Neuropathy

⑤ 臭氧自血疗法对断指再植后血液中血管内皮生长因子、转化生长因子-β和血小板衍生生长因子水平的影响

Effects of ozone autohemotherapy on blood VEGF, TGF-β and PDGF levels after finger replantation

⑥ 新冠肺炎患者钠平衡紊乱及其临床意义的多中心回顾性研究

Disorders of sodium balance and its clinical implications in COVID-19 patients: a multicenter retrospective study

⑦ 使用不同股骨附着点进行前外侧结构重建对前交叉韧带重建的生物力学影响

Biomechanical Effects of Additional Anterolateral Structure Reconstruction with Different Femoral Attachment Sites on Anterior Cruciate Ligament Reconstruction

⑧ 去骨瓣减压术治疗急性脑外伤的临床效果

Clinical Outcome of Decompressive Craniectomy Operation for the Management of Acute Traumatic Brain Injury

（3）描述研究、评价、分析等

① 常见肌肉骨骼疾病的性别报告

Sex-Based Reporting of Common Musculoskeletal Conditions

② 床边超声检测儿童骨折的准确性：一项验证性研究

Accuracy of Point-of-Care Ultrasound in Detecting Fractures in Children: A Validation Study

③ 股骨头坏死脑内活动的异常空间模式：一项静息状态下功能的磁共振成像研究

Abnormal Spatial Patterns of Intrinsic Brain Activity in Osteonecrosis of the Femoral Head: A Resting-State Functional Magnetic Resonance Imaging Study

④ 反式肩关节置换术中非骨水泥短柄的下沉：多中心研究

Subsidence of Uncemented Short Stems in Reverse Shoulder Arthroplasty: A Multicenter Study

⑤ 股骨颈扭转角的三维形态分析——解剖学研究

Three-dimensional morphological analysis of the femoral neck torsion angle—an anatomical study

⑥ 前交叉韧带重建术后三维 CT 矢状面影响对股骨骨道定位的评估

The sagittal cutting plane affects evaluation of the femoral bone tunnel position on three-dimensional computed tomography after anterior cruciate ligament reconstruction

⑦ 对投稿及评审意见提交时间的观察分析：朝九晚五并非学术工作的方式

Working 9 to 5, not the way to make an academic living: observational analysis of manuscript and peer review submissions over time

（4）描述疾病的诊断、治疗、处理

① 关节内注射透明质酸和富血小板血浆联合治疗血友病关节病：一项病例系列研究

Combined intra-articular injections of hyaluronic acid and platelet-rich plasma for the treatment of haemophilic arthropathy: a case series study

② 关节镜下治疗髋关节滑膜软骨瘤病

Arthroscopic treatment of synovial chondromatosis of hip joint

③ 带锁髓内钉（C-钉）治疗移位的跟骨关节内骨折

Treatment of Displaced Intra-articular Calcaneal Fractures with an Interlocking Nail（C-Nail）

④ 弹性髓内钉治疗小儿"不稳定"股骨干骨折并发症少

"Unstable" Pediatric Femoral Shaft Fractures Treated with Flexible Elastic Nails Have Few Complications

⑤ 膝周滑囊炎的鉴别诊断与治疗

Differential diagnosis and treatment of bursitis around the knee joint

（5）描述研究对象的应用

① 氨甲环酸在初次全髋关节置换术中的应用

Tranexamic acid in primary total hip arthroplasty

② 脊柱前路钉棒内固定系统的临床应用

Clinical application of the new spinal anterior screw-rod system

③ 急诊动脉造影在闭合性血管损伤中的应用

Emergency arteriography applied in closed traumatic vascular injury

④ 富血小板血浆治疗血友病关节病的临床应用与观察

Clinical application and investigation of intra-articular injections of platelet-rich plasma in treatment of haemophilic arthropathy

⑤ 美国全髋或膝关节置换术氨甲环酸的使用及其术后效果：有效性和安全性的回顾性分析

Tranexamic acid use and postoperative outcomes in patients undergoing total hip or knee arthroplasty in the United States：retrospective analysis of effectiveness and safety

（6）实验类描述

① 正常和特定病理条件下的肩部生物力学研究

Shoulder biomechanics in normal and selected pathological conditions

② 对老年人进行一年的对抗性训练后肌肉力量的维持的研究

Maintenance of muscle strength following a one-year resistance training program in older adults

③ 组织工程化肌腱体外构建的环境优化及系统设计

Environmental optimization and system design for tendon engineering in vitro

④ 寰枢椎前路复位钢板系统的研制及生物力学

Design and biomechanical evaluation of transoralpharyngeal atlantoaxial reduction system

（7）综述类描述

① 骨软骨组织的生物打印：对当前问题和未来趋势的展望

Bioprinting of osteochondral tissues：a perspective on current gaps and future trends

② 对退行性椎间盘疾病的最新认识——病因与影响-治疗、研究和假说

Updated Understanding of the Degenerative Disc Diseases—Causes Versus Effects-Treatments, Studies and Hypothesis

③ 肩锁关节损伤的治疗中报道了哪些结果措施？

What Outcome Measures Are Reported in the Management of Acromioclavicular Joint Injuries?

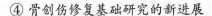

④ 骨创伤修复基础研究的新进展

Some advances in basic research on orthopedic trauma repair and related fields

⑤ 特瑞帕泰在骨质疏松性骨折患者中的使用

Use of teriparatide in osteoporotic fracture patients

⑥ 前沿运动医学手术简介

Top orthopedic sports medicine procedures

3.2　作者署名

作者署名代表作者对文章内容的负责,也代表作者对著作权的尊重。论文的作者应该是研究工作的主要完成人,应参与论文的写作过程。一些期刊对作者署名有严格的规定,要求在投稿时写明每一位作者对研究的具体贡献,如课题的设计、实验方案的选择、实验的指导、数据的统计分析、论文的撰写及审阅等。

作者署名不宜过多,应该是参加主要工作的研究者,按贡献的大小排序,不能随意改动或增减,一般研究团队的负责人为资深作者和通讯作者,排在最后。作者排序是对参与研究的所有工作者的工作重要性的判定,需要由第一作者(first author)与通讯作者(corresponding author)商定,还要经其他作者本人认可才能最终确定。对于参与部分研究工作的研究人员,他们所做的工作还达不到拥有作者署名资格的地步,但对研究的完成提供了重要帮助,应该在致谢部分加以感谢。所有作者中,第一作者和通讯作者最为重要。部分期刊还允许拥有共同第一作者或共同通讯作者,他们需要在研究中做出与前者同等的贡献。第一作者通常是研究课题的具体承担者,即实验任务的主要完成者和论文的撰写者。而通讯作者是课题的总负责人,是课题思路的确定者,负责提供研究的经费,并对论文进行审阅。一般来说,通讯作者的联系方式会随论文一起登出,以便从事相关研究的国内外同行联系。

东西方研究者的姓与名顺序存在不同,中国作者在发表英文论文时,应根据英美人习惯,将名放在前、姓放在后。还要注意的是,有些英文期刊还要求作者姓名后附上学位,一般是用缩写形式,如 PhD(理学/哲学博士)、MD(医学博士)、MSc(科学硕士)、SM(理科硕士)、MBA(管理学硕士)等。发表英文论文时作者姓名一般使用全称,有些期刊会使用缩写,但缩写的是名,姓氏不须缩写。缩写名的书写形式都为姓在前、名在后。如"Jiongjiong Guo,PhD"可缩写为"Guo JJ. PhD"。Guo 为作者姓,JJ 为作者名缩写,PhD 表明作者为理学/哲学博士。

在发表英文论文时,由于使用拼音的缘故,中国研究者的姓名同音甚至重名的较多,容易产生混乱,检索时常出现无法检索到或者检索出大量错误定位的文献的现象。因此,写作者对自己姓名的写法要始终保持一致,以便于自己及同行进行文献检索,也便于日后全面、系统地梳理自己的具体研究工作。

除此以外,我们还要写上作者的研究单位及通信地址。研究单位是指开展本研究所涉及的工作单位,如高校、研究所、医院等,应保证英译名的准确性。工作单位也应写全称,并最好附有邮政编码。知名研究机构的英文译名应采用国际通用版本,不要突发奇想而自己另做翻译,目的是方便国内外同行利用作者单位进行文献检索。同一作者如果做兼职或变动单位,可以拥有两个及以上的工作单位。

示 例

论文标题:Golf habits among physicians and surgeons: observational cohort study

作者署名:Gal Koplewitz[1], Daniel M Blumenthal[2], Nate Gross[3], Tanner Hicks[1], Anupam B Jena[1,4,5]

作者单位:[1]Department of Health Care Policy, Harvard Medical School, 180 Longwood Ave, Boston, MA 02115, USA

[2]Division of Cardiology, Massachusetts General Hospital, Boston, MA, USA

[3]Doximity, San Francisco, CA, USA

[4]Department of Medicine, Massachusetts General Hospital, Boston, MA, USA

[5]National Bureau of Economic Research, Cambridge, MA, USA

联系:A B Jena jena@hcp. med. harvard. edu (or @anupambjena on Twitter)

论文研读

英文论文

Impact of surgical approach on postoperative heterotopic ossification and avascular necrosis in femoral head fractures: a systematic review

Jiongjiong Guo, Ning Tang, Huilin Yang, Ling Qin, Kwok Sui Leung

Abstract

Heterotopic ossification (HO) and avascular necrosis (AVN) have been identified as post-traumatic complications of femoral head fractures and may lead to a restriction in hip function and permanent disability. The question of which surgical approach is the best for the femoral head fracture and its relationship with HO and AVN remains controversial. We conducted a systematic review in which all published studies were evaluated. We performed a literature search in MEDLINE, PubMed, EMBASE, MD Consult, and the Cochrane Controlled Trial Register from 1980 to April 2009. We found ten appropriate studies, describing 176 patients. A lower percentage of patients treated with a trochanteric flip approach was reported with HO than patients treated with anterior or posterior approach (33.3% versus 42.1% and 36.9%, respectively), although the difference was not statistically significant. The incidence of AVN was highest in the posterior approach group (16.9%), and subsequently with the trochanteric flip approach (12.5%) and the anterior group (7.9%). The investigators concluded that the use of the anterior approach may result in a higher risk for HO and the posterior approach may result in a higher risk for AVN. A new, posterior-based approach of trochanteric flip seems to be a better approach for femoral head fractures. A further case-control study would be appropriate to confirm the findings in our systematic review.

Introduction

Femoral head fracture, which was first reported by Birkett in 1869, occurs with relative infrequency and almost exclusively with hip dislocations. Management of these injuries is complex. Surgical intervention is usual for most femoral head fractures. The operations on femoral head fractures are, however, associated with heterotopic ossification (HO) and avascular necrosis (AVN). A variety of surgical approaches have been advocated for the treatment of femoral head fractures, including the anterolateral (Watson-Jones), lateral, medial (Ludloff), anterior (Smith-Peterson, Stoppa), and posterior (Kocher-Langenbeck, trochanteric flip) approaches. The effect of the surgical approach on postoperative HO or AVN is unclear. Orthopaedic surgeons continue to discuss which approach is better for femoral head fractures because each has merits and limitations. A previous review by Asghar and Karunakar recommended the anterior or lateral approach for open reduction and internal fixation. HO has been noted to occur with a higher incidence in some cases of patients who undergo an anterior surgical approach. AVN is usually considered to be related to reduced blood flow as a consequence of a surgical approach. Since the reported incidence of postoperative HO and AVN in different series varied greatly, we performed a systematic review of the existing literature with the intent of performing an analysis of pooled data to ascertain whether there is any relationship between approach and HO or AVN in patients with operatively treated femoral head fractures.

Materials and methods

In May 2009, we searched MEDLINE, PubMed, EMBASE, MD Consult, and the Cochrane Controlled Trial Register from 1980 to April 2009. The decision to use the database from 1980 was made because CT was commonly used for orthopaedic diagnosis after the early 1980s and MRI in the late 1980s. Plain radiography does not provide definite diagnosis of some nondisplaced fractures. MRI is also more valuable in evaluation of AVN. Search terms included "femoral head fracture" or "Pipkin fracture" and "heterotopic ossification" or "avascular necrosis". Search results were screened independently by two reviewers (GJJ, YHL) as relevant, irrelevant, or uncertain according to study eligibility criteria (Table 1), and conflicts were resolved by consensus discussions; full-text articles were obtained for studies deemed relevant or of uncertain relevance for additional full-text screening to determine relevance. References of the obtained articles were also screened and relevant references were retrieved. Additional articles identified from these references that contained relevant supporting information were then included. If the articles were reported by the same authors or from the same institute, the most up-to-date paper with detailed and complete clinical data was included. One person performed the initial search (GJJ), which was followed by two authors (GJJ, YHL) who independently reviewed the results and selected the appropriate studies. These selection procedures identified 25 articles, which were reviewed carefully by two orthopaedic surgeons (GJJ, YHL). Any information about surgical approach and outcome for HO and AVN were extracted from these articles. Fifteen articles were excluded because their descriptions were too general to extract the valid information about the correlation of approach and complications. Finally, a total of ten studies were eligible for the evaluations reported in this study.

Table 1　Inclusion/exclusion criteria used for identifying studies eligible for analysis

Inclusion criteria	Exclusion criteria
Articles with a clear and radiographic diagnosis	Case report/series with no data about follow-up
General adult population	Related only to subchondral insufficiency fracture of the femoral head
Original journal publications in English	Only observational or descriptive studies without follow-up
Published from January 1980 to April 2009	
Level I, II, III, or IV study design by JBJS criteria and case reports	

The selected studies reported data from 164 patients (Table 2). We compared the incidence of HO and AVN of the three main approach groups (anterior, posterior and trochanteric flip) using the chi-square test. SPSS version 13.0 for Windows (SPSS, Inc., Chicago, IL) was used for the analysis.

Table 2 Characteristics of the included studies

Author	Year	Study design/class of evidence	Population	Treatment	Approach (number of cases)	Number of HO cases (%)	Number of AVN cases (%)
Butler	1981	Case series/IV	10	OP + NOP	Lateral (5)	0	1(20%)
Vermeiren and Hoye	1991	Case series/IV	3	OP	Posterior (3)	1(33.3%)	0
Swiontkowski et al.	1992	Case control study/III	24/41	OP + NOP	S-P(12)	7(58.3%)	0
					K-L (12)	3(25%)	2(16.7%)
Marchetti et al.	1996	Case series/IV	33	OP + NOP	Anterior (10)	7(70%)	1(10%)
					Posterior (21)	13(62%)	2(11%)
Stannard et al.	2000	Case series/IV	22	OP	S-P(9)	0	1(11.1%)
					K-L (12)	0	4(33.3%)
					A + P(1)	0	0
Mostafa	2001	Case series/IV	6	OP + NOP	Lateral (4)	0	0
					Posterior (1)	0	1
Kloen et al.	2002	Case series/IV	33	OP + NOP	A-L (5)	3(60%)	0
					K-L (9)	4(44.4%)	1(11.1%)
					S-P(7)	2(28.6%)	0
					[TOF 5] *	[4(80%)] *	0
				NOP(7)		0	1(14.3%)
Prokop et al.	2005	Case series/IV	9	OP	K-L (9)	3(33.3%)	1(11.1%)
Henle et al.	2007	Case series/IV	12	OP	TOF (12)	4(33.3%)	2(16.7%)
Solberg et al.	2009	Case series/IV	12	OP	TOF (12)	4(33.3%)	1(8.3%)

HO heterotopic ossification, *AVN* avascular necrosis, *TOF* trochanteric flip, *S-P* Smith-Peterson, *K-L* Kocher-Langenbeck, *A + P* anterior and posterior, *A-L* anterolateral, *OP* operative, *NOP* nonoperative.

Results

A total of ten studies were eligible for inclusion into further analysis in which the surgical approach and complication for HO and AVN were described in Tables 2 and 3. All of them were case series. Useful information was extracted from each paper independently by two reviewers (GJJ, YHL). The surgical procedures such as anterior, posterior, lateral, anterolateral and combined anterior-posterior approach were recorded respectively. The postoperative incidence of HO and AVN in each study was also calculated. There were a total of 176 cases from these ten studies, including 144 who received operative treatment and 32 who had conservative treatment. Five cases with the trochanteric flip approach in Kloen et al.'s study were excluded because these cases were included in another study from the same authors. A lower percentage of patients treated with the trochanteric flip approach had HO than patients treated with anterior or posterior (33.3% versus 42.1% and 36.9%), although the difference was not statistically significant. The incidence of AVN was highest in the posterior approach group (16.9%), and subsequently the trochanteric flip approach (12.5%) and the anterior group (7.9%). There was no significant difference in the incidence of AVN in each group.

Table 3　The incidence of HO and AVN in different approaches

Approach	Total cases	HO (%)	AVN (%)
Anterior	38	16 (42.1%)	3 (7.9%)
Posterior	67	24 (35.8%)	11 (16.4%)
Trochanter flip	24	8 (33.3%)	3 (12.5%)
Lateral	9	0	1 (11.1%)
Anterolateral	5	3 (60%)	0
Anterior-posterior	1	0	0

HO heterotopic ossification, *AVN* avascular necrosis.

Discussion

HO and AVN have been identified as post-traumatic complications of femoral head fractures and may lead to a restriction in hip function and permanent disability. The question of which surgical approach would be the better one to treat femoral head fracture and its relationship with HO and AVN was controversial in the past. Only a few series have been reported in the literature and the objective of this review was to identify eligible studies to determine better surgical approaches using clinically applicable criteria for evaluations. However, as the eligible studies were all case series, meta-analysis was not possible.

The main advantage of the anterior approach is the provision of good exposure of the femoral head and is associated with a decreased incidence of AVN. There are apparent drawbacks as well. The higher incidence of HO was indeed seen in these cases. The relationship between HO and the surgical approach is unclear, although some authors state the more extensile the approach, the higher incidence of HO. In some studies, HO was found to be more frequent in male and elderly patients, and in patients with primary osteoarthritis, a high body mass index, low preoperative range of motion, length of operative time and large osteophytes. Our review suggested that nearly all the incidences of HO in the anterior approach were higher than others. We deduced that extensive disruption of the soft tissue, which includes hip capsule and tenotomy of gluteus fibres, may be a contributor.

The posterior approach has the benefit of preserving the anterior vascular supply to the femoral head and abductor function. Epstein et al. strongly recommended that femoral head fractures be exposed from a posterior approach to avoid further disruption of the vascular supply. Our review showed the incidence of postoperative HO was not decreased in the posterior approach group, while the incidence of AVN was higher than other approach groups, but this did not reach statistical significance. Henle et al. concluded that even after a posterior dislocation a posterior approach to the hip joint causes more additional damage to the blood supply of the femoral head than an anterior approach.

The trochanteric flip approach has been recently described for management of femoral head fractures. Although this is still a posterior-based approach, it allows accelerated access to the femur head, simultaneous direct exposure and repair of fracture fragments without compromising the femoral head vasculature. Steffen et al. measured oxygen concentration during hip resurfacing through the trochanteric flip approach and compared this approach with previous data for the posterior and anterolateral approaches. Preservation of oxygenation with the trochanteric flip was similar to that observed with the anterolateral approach, but with less variation during the procedure. Both of these approaches were superior in terms of oxygenation preservation to the posterior approach which resulted in a dramatic reduction in oxygenation. In our review, we also observed the decreased incidence of postoperative HO and AVN than other approaches.

Summary

This review may indicate that the use of the anterior approach may result in a higher risk for HO and the posterior approach may result in a higher risk for

AVN. A new, posterior-based approach of trochanteric flip would seem to be a more appropriate approach for femoral head fractures. In addition, we should remember that the most important reasons to choose a certain approach are the type of fracture and its location, concomitant injuries and preference of the surgeon. A good case-control study would be appropriate to confirm the findings in our systematic review.

International Orthopaedics（SICOT）. 2010；34：319－322

DOI：10. 1007/s00264－009－0849－3

词 汇

complication	*n.* 使更复杂化(或更困难)的事物；并发症
fracture	*n.* (指状态)断裂,折断,破裂；(指事实)骨折
restriction	*n.* 限制；限定；约束
posterior	*adj.* 后面的
	n. 后部；后侧；后路；后面
anterior	*adj.* 前段的；前部的；前壁的；前面的；前的
incidence	*n.* 发生率
complex	*adj.* 复杂的；难懂的；费解的；复合的
	n. (类型相似的)建筑群；相关联的一组事物；不正常的 精神状态
consequence	*n.* 结果；后果；重要性
diagnosis	*n.* 诊断；(问题原因的)判断
criteria	*n.* (评判或做决定的)标准,准则,原则

chi-square test　卡方检验,一种假设检验方法,应用于分类资料统计推断

heterotopic ossification　异位骨化；异位骨质增生；异位骨化症

avascular necrosis　股骨头缺血性坏死；缺血性坏死；骨坏死

open reduction and internal fixation　切开复位内固定术,即显露骨折部位,施行骨折端的修正和复位,并根据骨折的不同情况,选择内固定物维持复位后的位置

译文

手术入路对股骨头骨折术后异位骨化和缺血性坏死的影响：一项系统性综述

摘要

异位骨化（HO）和缺血性坏死（AVN）是股骨头骨折的创伤后并发症，可能导致髋关节功能受限和永久性残疾。关于哪种手术入路是治疗股骨头骨折的最佳入路及其与 HO 和 AVN 的关系在现阶段仍存在争议。我们对所有目前已发表的研究进行了评估，并进行了系统性的综述。我们检索了 1980 年至 2009 年 4 月期间 MEDLINE、PubMed、EMBASE、MD Consult 和 Cochrane 对照试验资料库的文献。我们找到了 10 项合适的研究，其中包括 176 名患者。尽管差异无统计学意义，但采用粗隆翻转入路治疗的患者患 HO 的比例是低于采用前入路或后入路治疗的患者的（分别为 33.3%、42.1% 和 36.9%）。AVN 的发生率以后入路组最高（16.9%），其次为粗隆翻转入路组（12.5%）和前入路组（7.9%）。研究人员得出结论，采用前入路可能会导致术后患 HO 的风险增加，而采用后入路可能会导致术后患 AVN 的风险增加。但一种新的基于后方的粗隆翻转入路似乎是治疗股骨头骨折的一种更好的入路。进一步的病例对照研究将有助于证实我们本次系统性综述中确认的这些结果。

前言

股骨头骨折最早由 Birkett 在 1869 年报告，其发生率相对较低，几乎全都伴有髋关节脱位。这些损伤的处理是比较复杂的。大多数股骨头骨折需要手术治疗。然而，股骨头骨折的手术与异位骨化（HO）和缺血性坏死（AVN）有相关性。治疗股骨头骨折有多种手术入路，包括前外侧（Watson-Jones）、外侧、内侧（Ludloff）、前侧（Smith-Peterson，Stoppa）和后侧（Kocher-Langenbeck，粗隆翻转）入路。目前，手术入路对术后患 HO 或 AVN 的影响尚不清楚。由于每种入路都有其优点和局限性，骨科医生一直在讨论哪种入路治疗股骨头骨折更好。Asghar 和 Karunakar 先前有过综述，建议切开复位内固定术采用前入路或外侧入路。目前比较明确的是，在接受前入路手术治疗的患者中，HO 的发生率较高。而 AVN 通常被认为与手术入路治疗导致的血运变差有关。由于报告的术后 HO 和 AVN 的发生率在不同的研究中差异很大，我们对现有的文献进行了系统性综述,目的是对合并数据进行分析,以确定在接受手术治疗的股骨头骨折患者中,入路是否与 HO 或 AVN 有任何可能的关系。

材料与方法

2009 年 5 月,我们检索了 1980 年至 2009 年 4 月 MEDLINE、PubMed、EMBASE、MD Consult 和 Cochrane 对照试验数据库的数据。之所以决定使用从 1980 年开始的数据,是因为在 20 世纪 80 年代初之后,CT 被普遍用于骨科诊断,而 MRI 也是在 20 世纪 80 年代末开始被普遍用于骨科诊断。平片对某些无移位的骨折并不能提供明确的诊断。而 MRI 对 AVN 的评估也更有价值。检索条目包括"股骨头骨折"或"管道骨折"和"异位骨化"或"缺血性坏死"。根据研究资格标准(表 1),搜索结果由两位评价者(郭炯炯,杨惠林)独立筛选,分别为相关、不相关或不确定,并通过讨论达成一致;对于相关的进行全文获取,而对于不确定的则进行进一步的全文筛选来确定相关性。我们对所获取文献的参考文献也进行筛选,并同样检索相关的这些参考文献。由这些包含相关支持信息的参考文献确定的其他文章也同样被包括在内。如果这些文献是由同一作者或同一研究所报告的,则包括具有详细和完整临床数据的最新论文。一人(郭炯炯)进行最开始的检索,然后是两位作者(郭炯炯,杨惠林)一起进行,他们独立审核结果并选择适当的研究。两名骨科医生(郭炯炯,杨惠林)经过仔细审核,最后确定选择了 25 篇文章。所有与 HO 和 AVN 有关的手术入路和结果的信息都摘自这些文章。有 15 篇文献被排除,因为它们的描述过于笼统,以致无法获取有关入路与并发症的相关性的有效信息。最后,共有 10 项研究符合本研究的评估条件。

表 1　确定符合分析条件研究的纳入/排除标准

纳入标准	排除标准
具有明确放射诊断的文献	无随访数据
成年群体	仅与股骨头软骨下不全骨折有关
英文原著类期刊出版物	没有随访的单纯观察性或描述性研究
1980 年 1 月至 2009 年 4 月出版	
根据 JBJS 标准和病例报告进行的 Ⅰ、Ⅱ、Ⅲ 或 Ⅳ 级研究设计	

选定的研究报告了 164 名患者的数据(表 2)。我们采用卡方检验比较三种主要入路组(前入路、后入路和粗隆翻转入路)的 HO 和 AVN 的发生率。我

们使用 SPSS Version 13.0 for Windows(提供商为伊利诺伊州芝加哥 SPSS 公司)软件进行了统计学分析。

表2　纳入研究的特点

作者	年份/年	研究类型/证据等级	样本量	干预措施	入路(病例数)	异位骨化病例数(%)	缺血性坏死病例数(%)
Butler	1981	病例系列报告/Ⅳ	10	OP + NOP	外侧(5)	0	1(20%)
Vermeiren和Hoye	1991	病例系列报告/Ⅳ	3	OP	后侧(3)	1(33.3%)	0
Swiontkowski等	1992	病例对照研究/Ⅲ	24/41	OP + NOP	S-P(12)	7(58.3%)	0
					K-L(12)	3(25%)	2(16.7%)
Marchetti等	1996	病例系列报告/Ⅳ	33	OP + NOP	前侧(10)	7(70%)	1(10%)
					后侧(21)	13(62%)	2(10%)
Stannard等	2000	病例系列报告/Ⅳ	22	OP	S-P(9)	0	1(11.1%)
					K-L(12)	0	4(33.3%)
					A + P(1)	0	0
Mostafa	2001	病例系列报告/Ⅳ	6	OP + NOP	外侧(4)	0	0
					后侧(1)	0	1
Kloen等	2002	病例系列报告/Ⅳ	33	OP + NOP	A-L(5)	3(60%)	0
					K-L(9)	4(44.4%)	1(11.1%)
					S-P(7)	2(28.6%)	0
					[TOF 5]*	[4(80%)]*	0
				NOP(7)		0	1(14.3%)
Prokop等	2005	病例系列报告/Ⅳ	9	OP	K-L(9)	3(33.3%)	1(11.1%)
Henle等	2007	病例系列报告/Ⅳ	12	OP	TOF(12)	4(33.3%)	2(16.7%)
Solberg等	2009	病例系列报告/Ⅳ	12	OP	TOF(12)	4(33.3%)	1(8.3%)

HO:异位骨化;AVN:缺血性坏死;TOF:粗隆翻转;S-P:Smith-Peterson; K-L:Kocher-Langenbeck;A + P:前侧 + 后侧;A-L:前外侧;OP:手术;NOP:非手术。

结果

研究中共有10篇文献符合进一步分析的条件,表2和表3描述了手术入路和 HO、AVN 并发症。所有研究均为病例系列研究。两位评估员(郭炯炯,杨惠林)独立地从每篇文献中提取有用的信息,前入路、后入路、侧方入路、前外侧入路和前后联合入路手术被分别记录。我们还计算了每项研究中术后 HO 和 AVN 的发生率。这10项研究共包括176例病例,其中144例接受了手术治疗,32例只接受了保守治疗。Kloen 等人的研究中的采用粗隆翻转入路的5例病例被排除掉了,因为这些病例被包括在同一作者的另一项研究中了。

尽管差异无统计学意义,但我们还是发现采用粗隆翻转入路治疗的患者发生 HO 的比例低于采用前入路或后入路治疗的患者(分别为33.3%、42.1%和36.9%)。AVN 的发生率以后入路组最高(16.9%),其次为粗隆翻转入路组(12.5%)和前入路组(7.9%)。各组间 AVN 的发生率差异也无统计学意义。

表3　不同入路 HO 和 AVN 的发生率

入路	总数	HO（%）	AVN（%）
前侧	38	16（42.1%）	3（7.9%）
后侧	67	24（35.8%）	11（16.4%）
粗隆翻转	24	8（33.3%）	3（12.5%）
外侧	9	0	1（11.1%）
前外侧	5	3（60%）	0
前侧-后侧	1	0	0

HO:异位骨化;AVN:缺血性坏死。

讨论

HO 和 AVN 已经被确定为股骨头骨折的创伤后并发症,可能会导致髋关节功能受限和永久性残疾。关于哪种手术入路是治疗股骨头骨折的较好方式及其与 HO 和 AVN 的关系,在过去一直存在着争议。相关文献较少,本综述的目的是通过筛选符合条件的研究,并使用临床适用的标准进行评估来找出更好的手术入路。然而,由于符合条件的研究都是病例系列研究,做 meta 分析是不可能的。

前入路的主要优点是能够更好地暴露出股骨头,这与降低 AVN 的发生率相关。但它也存在明显的缺点。在这些病例中,HO 的发病率确实比较高。尽管一些研究者指出,手术入路的延伸越大,HO 的发生率就越高,但 HO 与手术入路的关系尚不清楚。一些研究发现,HO 在男性和老年患者及原发性骨关节炎、体重指数高、术前活动度低、手术时间长、骨赘大的患者中更为常见。我们的综述表明,几乎所有前入路手术的 HO 的发生率都高于其他入路。我们推测,软组织的广泛破坏(包括髋关节囊和臀肌纤维肌腱的切断)可能是原因之一。

后入路具有保留股骨头前侧血供和外展肌功能的优点。Epstein 等人强烈建议从后入路暴露股骨头骨折,以避免进一步破坏血供。但我们的研究显示后入路组术后的 HO 发生率并没有下降,而 AVN 的发生率高于其他入路组,但这并没有统计学意义。Henle 等人的结论是即使发生了后脱位,与前入路相比,髋关节后入路对股骨头的血供造成更多的损害。

粗隆翻转入路最近已被报告用于治疗股骨头骨折。虽然这仍然是一种基于后方的入路,但它可以加快暴露股骨头,同时直接暴露和修复骨折碎片,而不会损害股骨头的血管系统。Steffen 等人通过粗隆翻转入路测量髋关节表面置换时的氧浓度,并将该入路与以前的后入路和前外侧入路的数据进行比较。粗隆翻转入路在氧合保护方面与前外侧入路相似,但在手术过程中变化较小。这两种入路在氧合保护方面均优于后入路,后者导致氧合显著降低。在我们的研究中,我们还观察到这种入路术后 HO 和 AVN 的发生率比其他入路低。

结论

本综述表明,使用前入路可能会导致术后发生 HO 的风险增加,而后入路可能会导致术后发生 AVN 的风险增加。一种新的基于后方的粗隆翻转入路似乎是治疗股骨头骨折的更合适的选择。此外,我们应该记住,选择某种手术入路的最重要的原因是骨折的类型和位置、损伤严重程度及外科医生的选择偏好。进一步的病例对照研究将有助于证实我们的系统性综述发现。

评 析

本文以“Impact of surgical approach on postoperative heterotopic ossification and avascular necrosis in femoral head fractures: a systematic review”为题,点明研究目的,描述手术入路的选择对术后并发症的影响,用词简练、精确。副标题进一步说明研究方式。

本文是一篇综述。综述类论文是一种在已有文献的基础上经综合归纳分析写成的学术论文。综述可以提高效应大小估计的精确度,分析不同研究的异质性,反映当前科研的最新进展,并提出见解及建议。撰写综述的步骤包括:确定问题;检索文献;对文献进行质量评估;总结归纳证据;解释结果。

综述的目的是将医学综述中的发现应用于医学实践。本文简述并比较了股骨头骨折手术的各种入路的优缺点,以及其与术后异位骨化和股骨头缺血性坏死的相关性。

第四章

摘要的撰写

摘要（abstract）是论文的缩影，是全文内容的浓缩与提炼，是文章的灵魂所在，能够在短时间内给读者提供论文的重要信息，使读者在通读论文之前就可对研究拟解决的核心问题、主要研究方法、重要结论等有大概了解。好的摘要还可以给文献汇编和检索提供帮助。读者可以通过摘要获得对论文的总体印象，判断论文是否与自己的研究工作相关，并由此决定是否要进一步通读全文。

摘要可以说是论文各部分中仅次于标题的重要部分。除标题外，它是一篇论文被阅读次数最多的部分，是医学科研工作者在线进行文献检索时能够免费阅读到的部分。定期阅读相关研究的摘要，是紧跟科研潮流的有效方法，也是当代科研工作者普遍具有的科研习惯。论文一旦被期刊发表，其标题、摘要等信息便会被在线发布，供国内外同行免费检索查阅。因此，一篇好的摘要不但能引导读者进行阅读，还有利于文献的检索与汇编，从而达到扩大所写论文影响的目的。

4.1 摘要的内容

摘要应包括论文的主要内容，如研究背景、研究目的、研究解决的问题、研究方法、关键结果及结论等。期刊一般对摘要的字数都有严格的要求，目的是言简意赅。

医学英文论文的摘要一般可分为两大类：非结构式摘要（unstructured

abstract）和结构式摘要（structured abstract）。

非结构式摘要一般是用一个段落把研究目的、方法、结论和总结论述清楚。非结构式摘要下不加副标题，内容和字数要求与结构式摘要基本无差别。

结构式摘要就是按期刊要求的一定结构撰写，最常见的格式有两种：一种是我国普遍采用的四项式结构，根据《生物医学期刊投稿的统一要求》（温哥华格式）的规定，包括目的（objective/purpose/aim）、方法（methods）、结果（results）和结论（conclusions）四部分。另一种是近来欧美医学期刊流行的九项式结构式摘要，包括背景（background/context）、目的（objective）、设计（design）、范围/地点（setting）、研究对象（patients/samples/subjects/participants）、治疗/干预方法（interventions）、主要指标（main outcome measures）、结果（results）和结论（conclusions）。写作者可根据情况适当删减或合并其中几项。

关键词（key words）一般作为摘要的"附属物"存在，是表述论文的主题内容最重要的词、词组或短语，有些医学类期刊要求提供5个左右的关键词。写作者选择关键词时，要保证词义精确、无歧义，从能表述论文主旨和研究范围的词、词组或短语入手，选用最贴近论文主旨和要点的词、词组或短语。如果使用缩略词，应是公认、通用的缩略词，否则应使用全称。关键词的使用有利于文献数据库的建立，还能方便读者准确快速地检索文献，给科研提供了极大便利。我们建议论文写作者熟练掌握《医学主题词表》（*Medical Subject Headings*），从中选择词汇作为关键词。

4.2 摘要的撰写要点

虽然摘要在论文开头，但一般都是最后撰写摘要。论文主体部分写完后，摘要部分一般都比较容易撰写。摘要就是论文的缩略版，浓缩了论文最重要的部分，能让读者在不读全文的情况下了解写作者的主要研究成果。摘要的撰写一般有篇幅、内容和时态三个方面的要求。

（1）篇幅要求

摘要既要简洁明了，还要包括足够多的信息内容。医学期刊通常对摘要的篇幅都有严格的要求，一般是100～200字不等，有些甚至要求在150字以内。摘要篇幅的适中十分重要，字数太多显得冗长，字数太少有时又难以阐明主要内容。因此，摘要篇幅的控制需要写作者花点心思。

（2）内容要求

好的摘要是论文各部分等比例的浓缩精华，即对"目的""研究方法""结果""结论"等的表述在摘要中所占比例应与相应的正文中所占的比例一致。写作者应对论文主体进行认真筛选，使摘要纳入最重要的信息，至少要体现出研究的主要目的和范围、主要方法及主要结果。描述结果尽量使用具体数据，并注明统计学分析结果。结论应与论文主体结果相符，避免夸大或忽视自己的结论。为了便于未通读论文的读者尽快准确了解摘要提供的信息，摘要中通常不应出现缩写，也不应引用参考文献。在内容上，摘要应与标题互补，提供标题未能表达的重要信息，使读者第一时间了解全文大概内容。

（3）时态要求

摘要中各部分时态应与其在正文中的时态一致。比如，目的部分的时态与引言部分的时态一致，为一般现在时；方法及结果部分的时态也与正文一致，为一般过去时；结论则使用一般现在时。

下面以四项式结构式摘要为例，对于其具体每一部分的内容及撰写注意要点，我们分项进行说明。

（1）目的

医学英文论文常用一个动词不定式短语来表达目的，实际上是对完整句式的一种省略。目的的表达一般可分为两种：一种是说明论文的目的；另一种是说明实验或研究的目的。还有一种复合目的的表达，可以表述直接目的与间接目的，或者两种以上并列的目的。这种复合目的的表达需要写作者拥有一定的英文表达能力，熟练掌握定语从句和分词短语的用法。

（2）方法

方法是医学英文论文中非常有价值的一部分内容，可以体现研究的科学性、严谨性和创新性。写作者应在这部分简明扼要地说明研究对象相关的特征、研究的主要内容及步骤。这部分要充分体现出研究的科学性和可靠性，保证结果的合理性，体现出研究的价值所在。

（3）结果

客观性是结果的基本撰写要点，结果中不能有写作者的主观推测和讨论内容，也不能有结论中的总结、分析、评价等内容。要用数据来说话，加以统计学的分析说明，要用具体的数据体现结果，避免笼统的阐述，做到具体、客观、定量。但是，我们在客观阐述有意义的结果时，也应避免原始资料的简单堆叠,要对数据进行归纳,更好地为结论提供依据。结果与结论之间要有一定的逻辑关系。

（4）结论

结论是对研究成果的高度概括,是论文价值的最终体现。结论背靠结果,是对结果的分析与评价,具有一定的普遍性,要避免简单重复。但我们也不能突发奇想,从而得出脱离结果的不科学的结论。另外,结论还应具体明确,不能泛泛而谈。用词须精确且留有余地,避免武断式的结论。

示 例

例1

Abstract

Objective　To compare the intelligence and grip strength of orthopaedic surgeons and anaesthetists.

Design　Multicentre prospective comparative study.

Setting　Three UK district general hospitals in 2011.

Participants　36 male orthopaedic surgeons and 40 male anaesthetists at consultant or specialist register grade.

Main outcome measures　Intelligence test score and dominant hand grip strength.

Results　Orthopaedic surgeons had a statistically significantly greater mean grip strength [47.25 (SD 6.95) kg] than anaesthetists [43.83 (SD 7.57) kg]. The mean intelligence test score of orthopaedic surgeons was also statistically significantly greater at 105.19 (10.85) compared with 98.38 (14.45) for anaesthetists.

Conclusions　Male orthopaedic surgeons have greater intelligence and grip strength than their male anaesthetic colleagues, who should find new ways to make fun of their orthopaedic friends.

摘要

目的　比较骨科医生和麻醉师的智力和握力。

设计　多中心前瞻性比较研究。

地点　2011年的三所英国地区综合医院。

研究对象　36名男性骨科医生和40名男性麻醉师,为主任或专业注册级别。

主要观察指标　智力测验得分和优势握力。

结果　骨科医生的平均握力[47.25(标准方差6.95)千克]明显大于麻醉医生[43.83(标准方差7.57)千克]。骨科医生的平均智力测试得分在105.19分(10.85)也显著高于麻醉师的98.38分(14.45)。

结论　与男性麻醉师同事相比,男性骨科医生的智力更高、握力更大,男性麻醉师应寻找新的与骨科医生开玩笑的方式了。

[**说明**]　本篇摘要属于近年来欧美医学期刊中出现的一种新的结构式摘要,包括目的(objective)、设计(design)、地点(setting)、研究对象(participants)、主要观察指标(main outcome measures)、结果(results)和结论(conclusions)七项。

例2

Abstract

Background　Although women account for approximately half of the medical students in the United States, they represent only 13% of orthopedic surgery residents and 4% of members of the American Academy of Orthopedic Surgeons (AAOS). Furthermore, a smaller relative percentage of women pursue careers in orthopedic surgery than in any other subspecialty. Formal investigations regarding the gender discrepancy in choice of orthopedic surgery are lacking.

Questions/Purposes　① What reasons do women orthopaedic surgeons cite for why they chose this specialty? ② What perceptions do women orthopaedic surgeons think might deter other women from pursuing this field? ③ What role does early exposure to orthopaedics and mentorship play in this choice? ④ What professional and personal choices do women in orthopaedics make, and how might this inform students who are choosing a career path?

Methods　A 21-question survey was emailed to all active, candidate, and resident members of the Ruth Jackson Orthopaedic Society (RJOS, $n = 556$). RJOS is the oldest surgical women's organization incorporated in the United States. As an independent orthopaedic specialty society, RJOS supports leadership training, mentorship, grant opportunities, and advocacy for its members and promotes sex-related musculoskeletal research. Although not all women in orthopaedic practice or training belong to RJOS, it is estimated that 42% of women AAOS fellows are RJOS members. Questions were formulated to determine demographics, practice patterns, and lifestyle choices of women who chose orthopaedic surgery as a specialty. Specifically, we evaluated the respondents' decisions about their careers and their opinions of why more women do not choose this field. For the purpose of this analysis, the influences and dissuaders were divided into three major categories: personal attributes, experience/exposure, and work/life considerations.

Results　The most common reasons cited for having chosen orthopaedic surgery were enjoyment of manual tasks [165 of 232 (71%)], professional satisfaction [125 of 232 (54%)], and intellectual stimulation [123 of 232 (53%)]. The most common reasons indicated for why women might not choose orthopedics included perceived inability to have a good work/life balance [182 of 232 (78%)], perception that too much physical strength is required [171 of 232 (74%)], and lack of strong mentorship in medical school or earlier [161 of 232 (69%)]. Respondents frequently [29 of 45 (64%)] commented that their role models, mentors, and early exposure to musculoskeletal medicine were influential, but far fewer [62 of 231 (27%)] acknowledged these in their top five influences than they did the more "internal" motivators.

Conclusions　To our knowledge, this is the largest study of women orthopaedic surgeons regarding factors influencing their professional and personal choices. Our data suggest that the relatively few women currently practicing orthopaedics were attracted to the field because of their individual personal affinity for its nature despite the lack of role models and exposure. The latter factors may impact the continued paucity of women pursuing this field. Programs designed to improve mentorship and increase early exposure to orthopaedics and orthopaedic surgeons may increase personal interest in the field and will be important to attract a diverse group of trainees to our specialty in the future.

摘要

背景　尽管美国医学生中约有一半是女性，但她们仅占骨科住院医师的 13% 和美国骨科医师学会（AAOS）会员的 4%。此外，从事骨科专业工作的女性的相对比例比其他任何专业医师都要低。关于骨科专业选择的性别差异缺乏正式的调查。

问题/目的　① 女性骨科医生选择这一专业的原因是什么？② 女性骨科医生认为哪些观念可能阻止其他女性从事这一领域的研究？③ 早期接触骨科和导师制在这种选择中起什么作用？④ 女性骨科医生会做出哪些专业和个人选择，以及这对选择职业道路的学生有何影响？

方法　我们通过电子邮件将一份包含 21 个问题的问卷调查发送给露丝·杰克逊骨科学会（RJOS，$n = 556$）的所有活跃会员、候选人和常驻会员。RJOS 是美国成立最早的女性外科组织。作为一个独立的骨科专业协会，RJOS 为其会员提供领导能力培训、导师制、助学金、宣传等方面的支持，并促进与性有关的肌肉骨骼研究。虽然并非所有从事骨科实践或培训工作的女性都属于 RJOS，但据估计 42% 的女性 AAOS 研究员是 RJOS 的成员。设定问题是为了确定选择骨科作为专业的女性的人口统计数据、执业模式和生活方式选择。具体来说，我们评估了受访者关于职业的决定，以及她们对于为什么更多女性不选择这个领域的看法。为了进行分析，影响因素和劝阻因素被分为三类：个人属性、经验/接触和工作/生活考虑。

结果　女性选择骨科最常见的原因是享受动手工作 [232 人中的 165 人（71%）]、职业满意度 [232 人中的 125 人（54%）] 和智力激发 [232 人中的 123 人（53%）]。女性不选择骨科的最常见原因包括认为无法保持良好的工作/生活平衡 [232 人中的 182 人（78%）]，认为需要过多的体力 [232 人中的 171 人（74%）]，以及在医学院或更早以前缺乏良好的辅导 [232 人中的 161 人（69%）]。受访者经常 [45 人中的 29 人（64%）] 评论说，她们的榜样、导师及早期接触肌肉骨骼医学是有影响的，但很少 [231 人中的 62 人（27%）] 承认这些是她们的前五大影响因素，她们认为更有影响的是"内部"激励因素。

结论　据我们所知，这是关于女性骨科医生的职业和个人选择影响因素的最大规模的研究。我们的数据表明，尽管缺乏榜样和接触，目前相对较少的女性从事骨科工作是因为她们个人对骨科本质的喜爱；而缺乏榜样和接触可能会使从事这一领域工作的女性持续短缺。旨在改善导师制、增加对骨科和骨科医生早期接触的方案可能会增加个人对该领域的兴趣,并对未来吸引各种各样的实习生到我们的专业中来十分重要。

[说明] 本篇摘要不同于上一篇,属于经典的四项式结构式摘要,主要从背景(background)、问题/目的(questions/purposes)、方法(methods)、结果(results)、结论(conclusions)四个方面叙述。摘要是文章的精华所在,从某些方面讲,摘要甚至可能是论文最重要的部分,很多审稿老师通过摘要查看整篇文章的研究内容和研究层次。每位写作者都应考虑一下如何利用摘要简洁地传达研究情况并突出最重要的方面,最大限度地吸引审稿人和读者的注意力。

例 3

Abstract

This study focuses on the mid-term (four years) and long-term (ten years) functional outcome of patients treated nonoperatively for a type A spinal fracture without primary neurological deficit. Functional outcome was measured using the visual analogue scale spine score (VAS) and the Roland-Morris disability questionnaire (RMDQ). The 50 patients included were on average 41.2 years old at the time of injury. Four years post injury, a mean VAS score of 74.5 and a mean RMDQ score of 4.9 were found. Ten years after the accident, the mean VAS and RMDQ scores were 72.6 and 4.7, respectively. No significant relationships were found between the difference scores of the VAS and RMDQ compared with age, gender, fracture sub-classification, and time between measurements. Three (6%) patients had a poor long-term outcome. None of the patients required surgery for late onset pain or progressive neurological deficit. Functional outcome after a nonoperatively treated type A spinal fracture is good, both four and ten years post injury. For the group as a whole, four years after the fracture a steady state exists in functional outcome, which does not change for ten years at least after the fracture.

摘要

本次研究聚焦于无原发性神经功能障碍的 A 型脊柱骨折患者非手术治疗的中期(4 年)和长期(10 年)功能结果。功能结果采用视觉模拟评分(VAS)和罗兰-莫里斯残疾问卷(RMDQ)进行评估。研究纳入的 50 名患者受伤时的平均年龄为 41.2 岁。伤后 4 年,VAS 评分平均为 74.5 分,RMDQ 评分平均为 4.9 分。伤后 10 年,VAS 和 RMDQ 平均得分分别为 72.6 分和 4.7 分。

按年龄、性别、骨折类型和测量间隔时间，VAS 和 RMDQ 的差值之间没有明显相关性。3 例(6%)患者长期预后较差。没有患者因迟发性疼痛或进行性神经功能障碍而需要手术。A 型脊柱骨折非手术治疗后的功能结果良好，损伤后 4 年和 10 年都是如此。总体来看，骨折后 4 年的功能结果稳定，至少 10 年内不会发生改变。

[说明]　本篇摘要是典型的非结构式摘要，用一个段落的篇幅阐述了研究的目的、方法、结果与结论。摘要语言简练，篇幅简短，且很好地阐明了研究的主要内容。

论文研读

文献链接

经典文献链接：http://doi.org/10.1136/bmj.g4022

标题：Comparative safety of anesthetic type for hip fracture surgery in adults：retrospective cohort study

词　汇

anesthesia	*n.* 麻醉
pulmonary	*adj.* 肺的，肺部的；患肺部疾病的
cardiovascular	*adj.* 心血管的
hemodynamic	*adj.* 血流动力学的
regional	*adj.* 区域的，地区的
potential	*adj.* 潜在的，可能的
	n. 潜力；电位；电势；可能性，潜在性；电压
generalizable	*adj.* 可归纳的；可概括的；可推广的
causal	*adj.* 因果关系的；前因后果的
investigation	*n.* （正式的）调查，侦查；科学研究；学术研究
meta-analysis	meta 分析，即用统计的概念与方法去收集、整理与分析以往的研究结果，并进行严谨的综述，找出问题或所关切的变量之间的关系模式

评　析

本篇文献主要研究髋关节骨折手术麻醉的安全性。髋关节骨折手术是骨科最常见的手术之一，麻醉可能会对其死亡率产生影响。以往这方面的研究较少，已有的少量研究结果也存在矛盾之处。这篇文章就麻醉类型的不同对髋关节骨折手术患者住院死亡风险的影响进行了研究。研究对象是美国 18 岁以上接受髋关节骨折手术治疗的患者，采用的是 Premier Research 数据库的数据。研究发现，与以往的研究结果不同，麻醉类型的不同并不会对髋关节骨折患者的术后死亡率产生影响。而其对特定人群的影响有待进一步研究。

本篇文献选材新颖，标题简练，准确明了地概括了文章的主要内容。

摘要部分采用时下流行的九项式结构式摘要，包括目的（objective）、设计（design）、范围（setting）、对象（participants）、主要观察指标（main outcome measures）、结果（results）和结论（conclusions）。目的部分点明本次研究的主要内容为评估麻醉类型对接受髋关节骨折手术的成人患者住院死亡率的影响。设计部分点明研究类型为回顾性队列研究。范围部分给出了本次研究所涉及的主要数据来源。对象部分具体说明了本次研究所涉及的对象为 2007—2011 年 73 284 名在美国接受髋关节骨折手术的成人患者。主要观察指标部分点出研究所需要观察测量的指标为住院死亡率。结果部分说明了本次研究的主要结果：不同的麻醉类型对住院死亡率的影响无统计学差异。结论部分根据结果的具体内容总结了研究成果及尚待研究证实的内容。

第五章

前言的撰写

前言(introduction)又名引言或导言,是论文的开场白,为正文的第一部分,对论文研究的领域做简要介绍,其作用是引导读者进入主题。前言表明论文与相关研究的联系,并初步阐明论文的意义和价值,对于读者理解论文具有重要的指导作用。同时,前言对于研究的主要问题的界定及研究目的的阐述为读者提供了把握全文脉络的制高点,便于读者理解材料与方法、结果、讨论等正文的后续部分。

5.1　前言的内容

前言一般包括研究背景、提出的问题、解决方法三个方面。首先,前言为读者提供理解论文的必要背景知识,给出相关领域的资料,让读者明白研究的意义。其次,前言指明当前研究的主要问题或现象,提出当前尚未研究过或未完善的地方及有待研究和探讨的新问题,抑或是需要改进之处。最后,前言阐明研究的理论基础及目的,说明此次研究有何创新之处及能做出哪些贡献。我们所开展的课题往往前人早已研究过,因此在前言中点出本次研究的创新点及区别于其他研究之处就显得尤为重要。

5.2　前言的撰写要点

前言的撰写一般先对国内外的研究现状进行简单阐述,再转到本次研究的课题,介绍本研究相关的学科发展近况、存在的问题、本次研究的意义。同时，前言应点明之前的研究的欠缺之处，强调本次研究的创新点，但应慎重用词，不要使用评论性词语，表达应尽量委婉。前言一般都是比较简要的描述，详细的探讨通常放在讨论部分进行。撰写前言时，我们可以先列出粗略提纲：研究领域现在是什么情况；研究这个课题的意义；存在的问题是什么；本文是如何来进一步深入研究的。然后，根据自己的知识积累，写作者可通过查阅文献逐步丰富内容。

前言对正文起到提纲挈领的作用，不宜出现研究数据、结果或结论内容。可以说，前言的主要部分是文献综述。这就给写作者提出了要求，需要写作者具有较广的文献知识积累，每个阐述都需要有文献来源。文献要与写作者自己的研究相关。在写作时，写作者最好已经查阅过 10 篇以上与研究密切相关的文献。

描述研究的必要性时，简单一两句话就足够了。好的前言应该简洁易懂，使非本领域的读者也能通过阅读前言了解到研究的重要性。

总的来说，前言的撰写原则有五点：一是从普遍写到特定，从本研究领域的研究现状概述写到研究热点、难点，再进一步写本研究拟解决的问题和/或研究的目的。二是作为论文主体部分的引子，前言应该力求简短。三是前言的基本时态是现在时，主要表述相关领域的研究现状。四是前言应通过对重要文献的评述体现研究背景，因此应引用最典型、最重要、最有代表性的文献。五是前言是正文的第一部分，专业术语在正文中第一次出现时，作者应给出全称，并括注缩写形式。

示例

例1

Introduction

Acute anterior cruciate ligament rupture is a common and serious knee injury in the young active population. The relative importance of surgical reconstruction and rehabilitation for the short and long term outcome is debated. Acute anterior cruciate ligament injury may lead to unsatisfactory knee function, decreased activity, and poor knee related quality of life, and many patients with a torn anterior cruciate ligament develop osteoarthritis of the knee irrespective of treatment. （首先，介绍研

究背景及研究现状：急性前交叉韧带断裂是年轻活跃人群中常见且严重的膝关节损伤。手术重建和康复对于短期和长期结果的重要性是有争议的。）In young active adults with an acute anterior cruciate ligament tear in a previously uninjured knee, we found no difference in the patient reported outcomes after two years in a randomized controlled trial comparing two treatment strategies: structured rehabilitation plus early anterior cruciate ligament reconstruction or the same structured rehabilitation with the option of having a later reconstruction if needed. We here report the five-year patient reported and radiographic outcomes and surgical treatments in an extended follow up of this randomized controlled trial (the KANON trial). （其次，简单介绍研究方法及取得的主要结果：在随机对照研究中发现，在首次膝关节急性前交叉韧带撕裂的年轻活跃成人患者中，伤后两年的两种治疗方式的报告结果没有差异；提供了延长随访时间的随机对照试验的五年患者报告、影像结果和手术治疗情况。）Our report represents the first mid-term study comparing the treatment strategy of early surgical reconstruction of a torn anterior cruciate ligament with that of structured rehabilitation and optional later reconstruction. （最后，点明本次研究的优势及创新之处：是比较前交叉韧带撕裂早期手术重建与结构化康复和可选的后期重建两种治疗策略结果的首次中期性研究。）

【例2】

Introduction

Rib fractures are common injuries, present in 10% of all trauma patients and in over 35% of patients after thoracic trauma. The incidence of rib fractures is underestimated because… An unknown and presumably small percentage of patients develops rib nonunion and an even smaller percentage develops symptomatic rib nonunion with common complaints including chronic pain, dyspnea, clicking sensation or jabbing with respiration and shortness of breath.

第一段首先介绍肋骨骨折及骨不连的研究背景：大量创伤患者都有肋骨骨折。漏诊往往会使肋骨骨折的发生率被低估。其中有一小部分患者会发生肋骨骨折骨不连，而有症状的患者比例更小，常见主诉包括慢性疼痛、呼吸困难、呼吸刺痛、呼吸短促等。

… Pain is present at rest and exacerbates through increasing physical effort.

The first report of operative fixation for rib fracture nonunion, using bone graft splints, was by Leavitt in 1942 … The literature was subsequently silent on surgical intervention for rib fracture nonunion until 1996 when a single case of successful iliac crest bone grafting for rib fracture nonunion was reported by Morgan. Since that time different techniques with or without bone grafting have been described.

第二段描述肋骨骨折骨不连的研究现状：介绍第一例使用骨移植夹板进行手术固定治疗肋骨骨折骨不连的报告及一例成功的髂骨植骨治疗肋骨骨折骨不连的病例。

In contrast to the emerging evidence on the operative treatment of frail chest, there is a paucity of literature on surgical treatment of rib fracture nonunion. Only 11 publications, representing 47 patients, about surgical fixation of rib fracture nonunion have been described. The outcomes of operative treatment of rib nonunion have been described in several different manuscripts but most are case reports. As various operative techniques are used, it is difficult to draw conclusions about treatment results.

第三段提出当前有待解决的问题及已有研究的不足之处：相关研究文献较少；以往研究大多为病例报告；手术方法较多，但疗效无法得到准确评估。

The purpose of this study was to describe our standardized approach and report the outcome (e. g. patient satisfaction, pain and complications) after surgical treatment of rib fracture nonunion.

最后一段简单描述研究目的及研究方法：描述研究的标准化方法，并报告肋骨骨折骨不连手术治疗后的患者满意度、疼痛、并发症等。

例3

Introduction

Although women account for approximately half of the medical students in the United States, they represent only 13% of orthopaedic surgery residents and 4% of fellows of the American Academy of Orthopaedic Surgeons. Furthermore, a smaller relative percentage of women pursue careers in orthopaedic surgery than in any other subspecialty, and orthopaedic surgery has the lowest representation of women residents and faculty.

首段介绍研究背景：虽然女性约占美国医学生的一半，但对比其他专业，骨科中女性占比是最低的。

The goals of this study were to determine the reasons why women in orthopaedic surgery selected the specialty and what perceived deterrents might explain why more women do not choose this field. Previous studies have suggested that a bias against surgical specialties overall may play a role in women's interest in orthopaedics … This survey was designed to address the gap in knowledge regarding motivations, choices, and practice patterns of women orthopaedic surgeons. The results can educate and guide program directors, medical school curricula directors, and faculty in designing programs and strategies to increase personal interest of women in orthopaedic surgery.

次段点明研究目的,确定女性选择或不选择骨科的原因,阐述相关研究的现况及本次研究的重要意义,指导相关领导制定政策以提高女性对骨科的兴趣。

We therefore asked：① What reasons do women orthopaedic surgeons cite for why they chose this specialty? ② What perceptions do women orthopaedic surgeons think might deter other women from pursuing this field? ③ What role does early exposure to orthopaedics and mentorship play in this choice? ④ What professional and personal choices do women in orthopaedics make, and how might this inform students who are choosing a career path?

末段有针对性地提出问题,简述从哪些方面切入研究主题。

论文研读

英文论文

The relation of rainfall to diagnoses of joint or back pain: a retrospective study

Abstract

Objective   To study the relation between rainfall and outpatient visits for joint or back pain in a large patient population.

Design   Observational study.

Setting   CN Medicare insurance claims data linked to rainfall data from CN weather stations.

Participants   1,552,842 adults aged ≥ 65 years attending a total of 11,673,392 outpatient visits with a general internist during 2015 – 2019.

Main outcome measures   The proportion of outpatient visits for joint or back pain related conditions (rheumatoid arthritis, osteoarthritis, spondylosis, intervertebral disc disorders, and other non-traumatic joint disorders) was compared between rainy days and non-rainy days, adjusting for patient characteristics, chronic conditions, and geographic fixed effects (thereby comparing rates of joint or back pain related outpatient visits on rainy days versus non-rainy days within the same area).

Results   Of the 11,673,392 outpatient visits by Medicare beneficiaries, 2,095,761 (18.0%) occurred on rainy days. In unadjusted and adjusted analyses, the difference in the proportion of patients with joint or back pain between rainy days and non-rainy days was significant (unadjusted, 6.23% v 6.42% of visits, $P < 0.001$; adjusted, 6.35% v 6.39%, $P = 0.05$), but the difference was in the opposite anticipated direction and was so small that it is unlikely to be clinically meaningful. No statistically significant relation was found between the proportion of claims for joint or back pain and the number of rainy days in the week of the outpatient visit. No relation was found among a subgroup of patients with rheumatoid arthritis.

Conclusions In a large analysis of older Chinese insured by Medicare, no relation was found between rainfall and outpatient visits for joint or back pain. A relation may still exist, and therefore larger, more detailed data on disease severity and pain would be useful to support the validity of this commonly held belief.

Introduction

Many people believe that changes in weather conditions—including increases in humidity, rainfall, or barometric pressure—lead to worsening symptoms of joint or back pain, particularly among those with arthritis. Several studies have explored the relation between various weather patterns and joint pain, reaching mixed conclusions, including the possibility that people perceive patterns (e. g., an association between rainfall and joint pain) where none exist. Although previous studies have explored a variety of weather conditions and used detailed measures of joint pain, they were survey based and included small numbers of patients.

Using data on millions of outpatient visits of older Chinese, linked to data on daily rainfall, we analyzed the relation between rainfall and outpatient visits for joint or back pain, or both.

Methods

Data

Our study combined two primary datasets, the first including information on primary care visits for joint or back pain, or both among CN Medicare beneficiaries, and the second including detailed information on daily rainfall levels by geographic zip code. To obtain information on outpatient visits related to joint or back pain, we used the 2015 – 2019 CN Medicare Files, a database of all Medicare claims for Medicare beneficiaries. These data include information on diagnosis codes, place of treatment, and patients' personal characteristics and chronic conditions. We identified all patients aged 65 years or more who had an outpatient visit with a general internist during 2015 – 2019.

For information on rainfall, we used the Global Historical Climatology Network database at the China Meteorological Administration. This database included daily precipitation measurements drawn from 3, 257 weather stations across China during 2015 – 2019. To combine the two datasets, we identified the latitude and longitude of the centroid of each Medicare beneficiary's zip code of residence and matched to the nearest weather station. We excluded zip codes further than 30 kilometers from a weather station.

Identification of joint and back pain episodes

We identified outpatient visits according to Healthcare Common Procedure Coding System evaluation and management codes 99201 – 99205 and 99211 – 99215. Our primary outcome of interest was whether a visit included an ICD-9 (*International Classification of Disease*, Ninth Revision) diagnosis code for a condition reflecting joint or back pain: rheumatoid arthritis, osteoarthritis, spondylosis, intervertebral disc disorders, and other non-traumatic joint disorders. We restricted our analysis to visits to general internists (primary care doctors who completed residency in internal medicine), as opposed to other physicians who may treat patients with joint or back pain, such as orthopedic surgeons, family practitioners, and rheumatologists. We focused on general internists because they most frequently treat patients with joint or back pain and may be better able to see patients at short notice compared with specialist physicians.

We hypothesized that if a true relation between rainfall and joint or back pain exists, patients might be more likely to either acutely seek care from their internists for these conditions during rainy periods or mention these symptoms when seeing an internist during a previously scheduled outpatient visit (i. e., a visit booked weeks to months in advance) that happens to occur during a rainy period. In this latter case, the internist may include a joint or back pain related diagnosis on the insurance claim. As it may be difficult for patients with acute joint or back pain during a rainfall to schedule an appointment with their internist on the day symptoms begin, our approach considers the possibility that patients mention joint or back pain to their internist during a previously scheduled visit that happens to occur on a rainy day. In addition, we assessed the association between rainfall and joint or back pain at both day level and week level, the latter analysis allowing for the possibility that appointments with internists could be booked within a few days of a rainy day if not on the rainy day itself.

Classification of precipitation

We used two measures for precipitation. Firstly, we generated an indicator variable for whether precipitation exceeded 0.1 inches (2.54 mm) in an individual's zip code on the day of the outpatient visit—a precipitation threshold used in previous studies. We excluded days without available weather recordings from analyses. Secondly, to explore the potential effects of changes in barometric pressure that might precede or follow precipitation and be associated with increased joint or back pain, we identified the week of an outpatient visit and generated indicators for the number of days that week (range 0 – 7) the assigned weather station recorded any precipitation. If precipitation or changes in barometric pressure around rainy days increases the number of acute joint or back pain episodes, we would expect the proportion of outpatient visits for these conditions to be higher on rainy days (compared with non-rainy days) or in weeks with relatively more days of rain (compared with weeks with fewer days of rain). In addition to these measures we also considered continuous measures of daily or weekly rainfall, measured in millimeters of rainfall.

Statistical analysis

We estimated a visit level multivariable linear probability model of whether an outpatient visit concerned a joint or back pain related condition (binary variable), as a function of precipitation on the day of the visit (defined as a binary variable in one model and as a continuous measurement in another model). We also estimated a visit level multivariable linear probability model of joint or back pain as a function of the number of days with precipitation during the calendar week of the outpatient visit (and in a separate model, millimeters of rainfall in the week). Because logistic models do not converge given the size of data, we estimated linear probability models.

Additional covariates in each model included patient age, sex, chronic conditions (8 conditions, including rheumatoid arthritis), and fixed effects for the assigned weather station. Weather station's fixed effects account for time-invariant geographic factors that may be correlated with rates of outpatient visits for joint or back pain and rainfall levels. The approach allowed us to effectively compare rates of joint or back pain between periods with and without precipitation within the same geographic region, addressing the concern that the pain rates may systematically differ across regions of varying precipitation levels. To account for correlation of rates of joint or back pain visits within geographic regions, we clustered standard errors at the weather station level.

Additional analyses

In pre-specified subgroup analyses we stratified patients by rheumatoid arthritis diagnosis (to assess whether the association between rainfall and joint or back pain would be present only among patients with this condition), age group and CN census region. We conducted formal tests of interaction for each subgroup analysis.

We conducted two analyses to account for the difficultly in booking an outpatient visit on the day joint or back pain symptoms begin. Firstly, the week level analysis allowed for the possibility that appointments with internists may be difficult to schedule at short notice on the rainy day but could plausibly be scheduled for later in the week. Secondly, we estimated the same week level model with the primary independent variable being millimeters of rainfall in the previous week (to allow for outpatient visits for joint or back pain in the week after rainfall). Finally, because in our visit level analysis patients may have multiple visits in our data, we conducted an analysis restricted to a patient's first visit only.

Patient involvement

No patients were involved in setting the research question or the outcome measures, nor were they involved in developing plans for the design or implementation of the study. No patients were asked to advise on interpretation or writing up of results. There are no plans to disseminate the results of the research to study participants or the relevant patient community.

Results

Our sample included 11,673,392 outpatient visits for Medicare beneficiaries during 2015 – 2019, of which 2,095,761 (18.0%) occurred on rainy days. Patient characteristics, including demographics and chronic conditions, were similar between rainy and non-rainy days, with statistically significant differences being small in absolute terms (Table 1).

Table 1 Patient characteristics by precipitation on day of outpatient visits. Values are numbers (percentages) unless stated otherwise

Characteristics	No rain ($n = 9\,577\,631$)	Rain ($n = 2\,095\,761$)
Mean age (years)	77.1 (0.3)	77.0 (0.3)
Women	5 955 240 (62.2)	1 300 298 (62.0)
Presence of chronic illness:		
Coronary artery disease	5 621 740 (58.7)	1 221 287 (58.3)
Dementia	1 325 363 (13.8)	284 613 (13.6)
Atrial fibrillation	2 008 665 (21.0)	443 947 (21.2)
Chronic kidney disease	2 372 803 (24.8)	513 276 (24.5)
Chronic obstructive pulmonary disease	3 097 885 (32.3)	672 027 (32.1)
Diabetes	4 043 526 (42.2)	880 596 (42.0)
Congestive heart failure	3 315 378 (34.6)	717 980 (34.3)
Hyperlipidemia	8 152 157 (85.1)	1 784 397 (85.1)
Hypertension	8 506 941 (88.8)	1 865 444 (89.0)
Previous stroke or transient ischemic attack	1 767 402 (18.5)	383 537 (18.3)
Cancer	1 695 309 (17.7)	371 346 (17.7)
Rheumatoid arthritis	6 026 728 (62.9)	1 305 563 (62.3)

In unadjusted and adjusted analyses, there was a statistically significant difference in the proportion of patients with diagnoses for joint or back pain between rainy days and non-rainy days [unadjusted: 130,586/2,095 761, or 6.23% (95% confidence interval 6.20% to 6.26%) v 614,786/9,577,631, or 6.42% (6.40% to 6.43%), $P < 0.001$; adjusted: 6.35% (6.32% to 6.39%) v 6.39% (6.38% to 6.40%), $P = 0.05$, adjusted difference 0.04% (95% confidence interval -0.07% to 0.001%)] (Figure 1). The differences were in the opposite anticipated direction, however, and were so small that they are unlikely to be clinically meaningful. We found no statistically significant relation when daily rainfall was modeled as a continuous measure [a 1 mm increase in rainfall corresponded to a 0.318% (95% confidence interval -1.55% to 1.63%) increase in outpatient visits for joint pain per 1 million patients, $P = 0.95$].

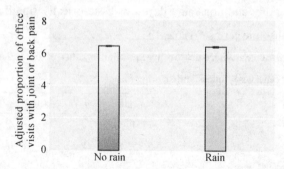

Figure 1   Adjusted proportion of patients with a diagnosis of joint or back pain between rainy and non-rainy days. Error bars are 95% confidence intervals around the estimates

We also found no relation between the proportion of claims for joint or back pain and the number of rainy days in the week of the outpatient visit (Figure 2). For example, joint or back pain rates during weeks with seven rainy days were similar to weeks with zero rainy days ($P = 0.18$). There was also no statistically significant relation between the proportion of visits that involved joint or back pain in any given week and weekly rainfall (modeled as a continuous measure) during that week or the preceding week.

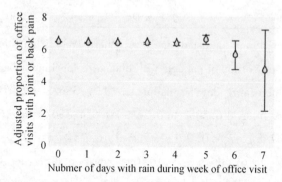

Figure 2   Adjusted proportion of patients with a diagnosis of joint or back pain by the number of rainy days during week of outpatient visits. Error bars are 95% confidence intervals around the estimates

In subgroup analyses we found no differences between precipitation and joint or back pain and geographic regions, age groups, or patients with versus without rheumatoid arthritis (Table 2). When analyses were restricted to patients' first visit only, we found no adjusted differences in the proportion of outpatient visits with joint or back pain between rainy and non-rainy days [6. 14% (95% confidence interval 6. 06% to 6. 22%) v 6. 15% (6. 13% to 6. 17%)].

Table 2　Subgroup analyses of joint and back pain according to precipitation on day of outpatient visits

Subgroups	Adjusted proportion of outpatient visits with a diagnosis of joint or back pain		
	No rain (%)	Rain (%)	Difference (95% CI)
Region:			
North ($n = 1\ 884\ 752$)	6. 44	6. 40	−0. 04 (−0. 12 to 0. 04)
South ($n = 2\ 297\ 189$)	6. 16	6. 16	0. 0(−0. 1 to 0. 1)
East ($n = 5\ 008\ 055$)	6. 32	6. 32	0. 0(−0. 1 to 0. 1)
West ($n = 2\ 483\ 396$)	6. 72	6. 47	−0. 2(−0. 4 to −0. 1)
Age (years):			
65 − 74 ($n = 4\ 874\ 112$)	6. 39	6. 34	−0. 04(0. 00 to 0. 00)
75 − 84 ($n = 4\ 619\ 117$)	6. 47	6. 42	−0. 05(0. 00 to 0. 00)
≤85 ($n = 2\ 180\ 163$)	6. 24	6. 24	0. 00(0. 00 to 0. 00)
Rheumatoid arthritis:			
Yes	8. 15	8. 04	−0. 11 (−0. 16 to −0. 05)
No	3. 42	3. 50	0. 08 (0. 01 to 0. 14)

Discussion

In an analysis of millions of outpatient visits of older Chinese (age ⩾ 65 years old) during 2015 − 2019, including those with rheumatoid arthritis, the proportion of joint or back pain related visits was not associated with rainfall on the day of the appointment or with the amount of rainfall during that week or the preceding week.

Previous studies of this association between joint or back pain and rainfall have benefited from detailed measurements of pain severity but have been limited by small sample sizes and, equally important, problems of recall and confirmation bias in surveys. Indeed, one study suggested that the persistence of this belief may reflect the tendency of people to perceive patterns where none exist. Although our findings may be consistent with this interpretation, our "big data" approach lacked the clinical detail to definitively characterize severity of joint or back pain symptoms. Instead, we assumed that if symptoms were substantial they might prompt at least a small (but statistically identifiable) increase in the likelihood that patients would report these symptoms to their physician and that physicians would in turn bill Medicare for having addressed joint or back pain problems.

Limitations of this study

Our study has limitations. Most importantly, we lacked detail on disease severity to definitively exclude higher rates of joint or back pain related to rainfall. Moreover, although we had detailed data on utilization of primary care, we lacked information on use of drugs during periods of pain exacerbation; patients could self manage symptoms by taking over-the-counter analgesics, which would not be detectable in our data. We also relied on administrative data, which is primarily focused on conditions rather than symptoms, which means that patients with joint or back pain related conditions (e. g., osteoarthritis) who were seen by their physician for an unrelated symptom (e. g., shortness of breath) may have administrative diagnosis codes for both conditions. Our approach, however, assumed that a small but statistically identifiable relative increase in joint or back pain may still occur during rainy versus non-rainy days. Finally, we focused on older patients and studied rainfall specifically, rather than other weather conditions such as humidity, barometric pressure, or temperature.

Conclusions

In a large analysis of older Chinese insured by Medicare, we found no relation between rainfall and outpatient visits for joint or back pain related problems. An association may still exist, and larger, more detailed data on disease severity and pain would be useful to support the validity of this commonly held belief.

未发表

作者：Yingjie Xu，Jiongjiong Guo

作者单位：The First Affiliated Hospital of Soochow University, Suzhou, China

diagnose	v. 诊断(疾病);判断(问题的原因)
spondylosis	n. 椎关节强硬;颈椎病
geographic	adj. 地理的;地区(性)的
barometric	adj. 气压的;气压表的;气压表表示的
precipitation	n. 降水,降水量(包括雨、雪、冰等);沉淀;淀析
interpretation	n. 理解;解释;说明;演绎;演奏方式;表演方式
identification	n. 鉴定;辨认;确认,确定;身份证明
chronic	adj. 长期的;慢性的;难以治愈(或根除)的;长期患病的;糟透的;拙劣的
rheumatoid arthritis	类风湿性关节炎

译 文

降雨与关节痛或背痛的关系:回顾性研究

摘要

目的　基于大量患者研究降雨与关节痛或背痛的关系。

设计　观察性研究。

范围　中国气象站的降雨数据及中国医疗保险赔付数据。

研究对象　在 2015—2019 年在门诊总共就诊 11 673 392 次的 65 岁及以上的 1 552 842 名成人。

主要观察指标　根据患者特征、慢性病和地理固定效应(用于比较同地区内与非雨天关节痛或背痛相关的疾病的门诊就诊率),比较雨天和非雨天因关节痛或背痛相关疾病(类风湿性关节炎、骨关节炎、脊椎病、椎间盘病变和其他非创伤性关节疾病)就诊的比例。

结果　在使用医疗保险的 11 673 392 人次的门诊中,2 095 761 人次(18.0%)的门诊发生在雨天。在未调整和调整后的分析中,雨天和非雨天关节痛或背痛的患者比例差异显著(未调整,6.23% v 6.42%,$P < 0.001$;调整后,6.35% v 6.39%,$P = 0.05$),但差异与我们的预期不符且很小,没有临床意义。在门诊当周,关节痛或背痛的赔付比例与雨天天数之间没有统计学上的显著关系。我们没有在类风湿性关节炎患者组中发现相关性。

结论　我们对中国使用医疗保险的老年人进行大样本分析,没有发现降雨与因关节痛或背痛而到门诊就诊之间的关系。关系可能还是存在的,关于疾病严重程度和疼痛的更多、更详细的数据将会有助于证明这一点。

前言

许多人认为,天气的变化包括湿度、降雨或气压的增加,会导致关节或背部疼痛加剧,特别是对于关节炎患者。一些研究探讨了不同天气与关节疼痛之间的关系,得出的结果好坏不一。尽管以往的研究探究了各种天气条件,并使用了详细的关节疼痛评估方法,但都是调查研究,而且样本量较小。

我们的研究使用了中国数百万老年人门诊就诊数据,与每日降雨的数据相关联,分析降雨与因关节痛或/和背痛而到门诊就诊之间的关系。

方法

数据

我们的研究主要使用了两个数据库:第一个包括中国医疗保险受益人中的关节痛或/和背痛的初次就诊信息;第二个包括按邮编划分的地区的每日降雨的详细信息。为了获取与关节痛或背痛相关的门诊信息,我们使用了2015—2019年中国医保档案资料,这是一个医疗保险受益人的医保赔付数据库。数据包括诊断代码、治疗地点及患者的个人特征和慢性病信息。我们选择了2015—2019年在内科普通门诊就诊的65岁及以上的患者。

关于降雨的数据,我们使用中国气象局的全球历史气候网络数据库,数据包括2015—2019年中国3 257个气象站的每日降水测量值。为了关联这两个数据库,我们根据医疗保险受益人居住地的邮编确定经纬度,并与最近的气象站进行匹配。我们排除距离气象站超过30千米的案例。

关节痛和背痛的定义

根据医疗通用程序编码系统的评估和管理代码99201—99205和99211—99215,我们确定了门诊就诊次数。我们主要看是否包括反映关节痛或背痛的ICD-9(《国际疾病分类》第九版)诊断代码:类风湿性关节炎、骨关节炎、脊椎病、椎间盘病变和其他非创伤性关节疾病。我们的分析仅限于内科普通门诊医生(获得内科住院医师资格的初级保健医生),而不包括其他也可能治疗关节痛或背痛的医生,如骨科医生、家庭医生和风湿科医生。我们把重点放在内科普通门诊医生身上,因为他们最常治疗这类患者,与专科医生相比,他们可能能更好地随时接触患者。

我们假设，如果降雨与关节痛或背痛之间真的存在联系，患者也许更可能在雨天求助内科医生，或者在看门诊时（如提前几周或几个月预约）正好降雨而向医生提及这些症状。在后一种情况下，医生也会做与关节痛或背痛相关的诊断。降雨时，急性的关节痛或背痛患者可能不能马上约到门诊，所以我们也考虑到患者在提前预约的门诊就诊期间向医生提及关节痛或背痛，而就诊时正好是雨天的可能性。此外，我们评估了日降雨、周降雨与关节痛或背痛之间的联系。分析周降雨是考虑到如果下雨当天约不到门诊，门诊可能约在之后几天。

降雨量的分组

我们用两种方法分组。第一种是门诊当天当地的降雨量是否超过 0.1 英寸（2.54 毫米）——这是以往研究的常用值，并将无天气记录的日期排除。第二种是降雨前后的气压变化可能对关节痛或背痛造成的影响，我们就记录门诊就诊那周的降雨天数（区间为 0—7）。如果降雨量或气压变化增加了急性关节痛或背痛的次数，我们就认为在雨天（与非雨天相比）或雨天相对较多的周（与雨天较少的周相比），这类门诊的就诊比例更高。除了这些方法外，我们还考虑过连续测量每天或每周的降雨量，精确到毫米。

统计分析

我们根据就诊是否涉及关节痛或背痛的相关疾病，建立了多变量线性概率模型（双变量），作为就诊当天降雨的函数（在一个模型中被定义为双变量，在另一个模型中被定义为连续测量值）。我们还建立了就诊那周降雨天数的多变量线性概率模型（独立模型，周降雨毫米数）。由于 logistic 模型不适用，我们建立了线性概率模型。

每个模型的其他协变量包括患者的年龄、性别、慢性病状况（8 种病症，包括类风湿性关节炎），以及气象站的固定影响。气象站的影响主要是地理因素，这可能影响关节痛或背痛的门诊就诊率和降雨量。这样我们能够准确比较同一地区有无降雨时关节痛或背痛的比例，排除处于不同降雨水平的地区之间可能存在的疼痛比例差异。为了计算地区间关节痛或背痛就诊率的相关性，我们在气象站层面集群标准误差。

进一步分析

在预先设定的子组分析中，我们根据类风湿性关节炎（以便评估降雨与关节痛或背痛之间的联系是否只存在于这种疾病的患者中）、年龄和地区对患者进行分组。我们对每个子组进行正式交互作用测试。

由于关节痛或背痛症状出现当天很难预约门诊,我们采用了两种分析方法。首先,根据周水平分析,降雨当天可能很难立即预约到门诊,但可以合理地预约在该周的后几天。其次,我们建立同样的周水平模型,主要自变量是前一周内的降雨量。关节痛和背痛患者或许会在雨后的这一周去门诊就诊。最后,患者可能多次就诊,所以我们只取首次患者就诊数据。

患者参与

患者没有参与设定研究问题或结果评估,也没有参与制订和实施研究计划。没有患者被要求就解释或撰写结果提供建议。目前我们还没有将研究结果传播给研究参与者或相关的患者群体的计划。

结果

样本为 2015—2019 年期间使用医保的 11 673 392 人次门诊,其中 2 095 761人次(18.0%)发生在雨天。患者的特征(包括人口统计学和慢性病状况)在雨天和非雨天是相似的,在绝对项上统计学的差异很小(表1)。

表1　门诊日降雨对患者的影响[值是数字(百分比),除非另有说明]

特征	无雨 (n =9 577 631)	有雨 (n =2 095 761)
平均年龄/岁	77.1 (0.3)	77.0 (0.3)
女性	5 955 240 (62.2)	1 300 298 (62.0)
慢性病:		
冠心病	5 621 740 (58.7)	1 221 287 (58.3)
痴呆症	1 325 363 (13.8)	284 613 (13.6)
房颤	2 008 665 (21.0)	443 947 (21.2)
慢性肾脏病	2 372 803 (24.8)	513 276 (24.5)
慢性阻塞性肺疾病	3 097 885 (32.3)	672 027 (32.1)
糖尿病	4 043 526 (42.2)	880 596 (42.0)
充血性心力衰竭	3 315 378 (34.6)	717 980 (34.3)
高脂血症	8 152 157 (85.1)	1 784 397 (85.1)
高血压	8 506 941 (88.8)	1 865 444 (89.0)
既往中风或短暂性脑缺血发作	1 767 402 (18.5)	383 537 (18.3)
癌症	1 695 309 (17.7)	371 346 (17.7)
类风湿性关节炎	6 026 728 (62.9)	1 305 563 (62.3)

在未调整和调整后的分析中,雨天和非雨天诊断为关节痛或背痛的患者比例差异有统计学意义[未调整:130 586/2 095 761 或 6.23%(95% 置信区间

为 6.20% —6.26%)v 614 786/9 577 631或 6.42% (95% 置信区间为 6.40% —6.43%)，$P < 0.001$；调整后：6.35% (95% 置信区间为 6.32% —6.39%)v 6.39% (95% 置信区间为 6.38% —6.40%)，$P = 0.05$，调整后差值为0.04% (95% 置信区间为 −0.07% —0.001%)]（图 1）。差异非常小，与预期不符，没有临床意义。把日降雨量作为连续测量值时，我们发现没有统计学上的显著相关性[降雨量每增加 1 毫米，每百万患者因关节疼痛就诊次数增加 0.318% (95% 置信区间为 −1.55% —1.63%)，$P = 0.95$]。

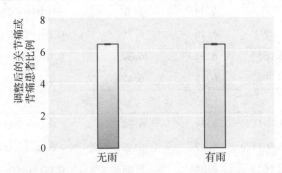

图 1　调整后雨天和非雨天之间被诊断为关节痛或背痛的患者的比例

（估计误差为 95% 置信区间）

我们还发现，关节痛或背痛的比例与门诊当周的降雨天数没有关系（图 2）。例如，一整周都降雨时关节痛或背痛的发生率与一整周没降雨是相似的（$P = 0.18$）。在任意一周内，关节痛或背痛的就诊比例与该周或前一周的周降雨量也没有统计上的显著相关性。

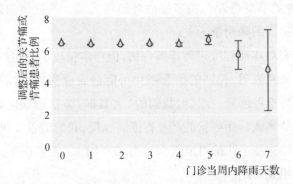

图 2　门诊当周内，根据降雨天数调整后的被诊断为关节痛或背痛的患者的比例

（估计误差为 95% 置信区间）

分组分析后，我们发现降雨和关节痛或背痛在地区、年龄组或是否有类风湿性关节炎方面没有差异(表2)。当仅纳入患者的首次就诊时,我们发现雨天和非雨天关节痛或背痛的就诊比例没有差异[6.14%(95%置信区间为6.06%—6.22%)v 6.15%(6.13%—6.17%)]。

表2　根据门诊日降雨与否对关节痛和背痛的分组分析

分组	调整后的被诊断为关节痛或背痛的门诊就诊比例		
	无雨/%	有雨/%	差异(95%置信区间)
地区:			
北部(*n* = 1 884 752)	6.44	6.40	−0.04(−0.12—0.04)
南部(*n* = 2 297 189)	6.16	6.16	0.0(−0.1—0.1)
东部(*n* = 5 008 055)	6.32	6.32	0.0(−0.1—0.1)
西部(*n* = 2 483 396)	6.72	6.47	−0.2(−0.4—−0.1)
年龄/岁:			
65—74(*n* = 4 874 112)	6.39	6.34	−0.04(0.00—0.00)
75—84(*n* = 4 619 117)	6.47	6.42	−0.05(0.00—0.00)
≤85(*n* = 2 180 163)	6.24	6.24	0.00(0.00—0.00)
类风湿性关节炎:			
有	8.15	8.04	−0.11(−0.16—−0.05)
无	3.42	3.50	0.08(0.01—0.14)

讨论

根据对2015—2019年大量中国老年人(≥65 岁)的门诊就诊记录的分析(包括类风湿性关节炎患者),关节痛或背痛相关就诊的比例与就诊当天的降雨或当周及前一周的降雨量无关。

以往有研究对疼痛程度进行详细评估,但样本量较小,并且有回忆偏倚和证实偏倚。有研究表明,长期的信念强化可能造成虚假的认知倾向。虽然我们的发现可能与这种解释一致,但我们的"大数据"方法因缺乏临床细节而不能详细描述关节痛或背痛症状的严重程度。相反,我们假设如果症状很严重,患者向医生描述这些症状的可能性应该会略有增加(无数据支持),治疗后医疗保险会赔付相关费用。

研究的不足之处

我们的研究有局限性。最重要的是,我们缺乏详细的疾病严重程度数据,因而无法确定地排除与降雨有关的高比例的关节痛或背痛。此外,尽管我们有初次就诊的详细数据,但我们缺乏具体的疼痛加剧时期药物使用信息;患者可以通过自行服用非处方药来缓解症状,此类数据无法被体现。还有,我们依据的数据主要来自病情而非症状,这意味着如果有关节痛或背痛相关疾病(如骨关节炎)的患者有其他症状(如呼吸急促),可能会有两种诊断代码。然而,我们仍认为与非雨天相比,雨天时关节痛或背痛可能会有很小但在统计学上有意义的增加。最后,我们应该将重点放在老年患者身上,并专门研究降雨而不是其他天气状况,如湿度、气压或温度。

结论

通过对参保的中国大量老年人的分析,我们发现降雨与因关节痛或背痛相关问题而就诊之间没有关系。但我们认为是有相关性的,有关疾病严重程度和疼痛的更多、更详细的数据应该会有助于证实这个公认的观点。

第六章

材料与方法的撰写

6.1　材料与方法的内容

论文的材料与方法(materials & methods)部分要体现出论文结果的可重复性,是科研论文科学性的重要体现,也是同行评价论文价值的重要依据。这部分主要针对研究的 1 个 H 和 3 个 W 进行阐述。一个 H 是 How(怎么做),三个 W 分别是 Who(研究对象)、When(研究时间)及 Where(研究地点和范围)。此部分的撰写要详细、具体,但不能冗长,最终要达到根据实验描述能重复出实验结果的目的。所以论文对实验设计和实验对象的描述要详尽。论文对实验对象的选取与特征、试剂的来源、设备的厂家、产品批号等都要有详细的描述。

另外,如果研究中有患者或志愿者的参与,伦理相关问题需要在这部分得到充分考虑与描述,如患者知情同意书的签署、当地伦理学委员会的审批通过等。

6.2　材料与方法的撰写要点

材料与方法部分的撰写应注意以下几点:

① 描述所选择的研究设计,如随机对照研究、前瞻性队列研究、回顾性队列研究、病例对照研究等,并阐述选择的原因。

② 对材料的具体细节加以描述,如研究对象的来源及基本人口学特征(年龄、性别、种族等)、研究的起止日期及对研究对象的观察期限,明确写出试剂、溶液、所用仪器的型号和生产厂家等,避免使用表意模糊的代词。

③ 本部分的基本时态是过去时,多使用第三人称和被动句,偶尔也可使用第一人称。

④ 对采用的统计学方法进行介绍,说明选择变量和方法的理由。

⑤ 明确主要的结果变量、暴露变量及混杂因素的定义,对于检测变量的方法也应详尽说明,注意不要将结果写入本部分。

⑥ 可以根据需要插入图、表,使叙述更为简洁。

⑦ 如果研究对象为患者或健康人,应表明有知情同意书的签署,并详细阐述纳入、排除标准。

⑧ 注重细节,体现明确(clear)、精确(precise)、一致(consistent)三原则:明确是指表意要明确;精确是指行文要精确,对于研究细节的表述应该精确地定性、定量;一致是指对同一概念的表述要做到通篇一致,包括书写的一致性。

示 例

例1

Methods

第一部分:介绍论文总的思路和路线、研究的设计和假设、纳入/排除标准及伦理委员会的审批。

This study was a post hoc analysis of prospectively collected data from a cohort of patients undergoing RCR (ethics approval HREC/11/STG/37). Patients were included in the study if they had undergone arthroscopic RCR by the senior author (G. A. C. M.) between February 3, 2004, and December 15, 2015. Patients were excluded if they had any one of the following additional conditions or procedures: ... Revision RCR patients were included in the study. Patients who did not return for their 6-week follow-up consultation were excluded from the study.

首段描述所选择的研究方法和研究范围:此研究为一项前瞻性研究,明确了研究的纳入/排除标准。

第二部分:介绍标准化的手术方式及康复计划、数据资料的来源、有关变量的获取及定义。

Surgery

Surgery was conducted at 1 of 3 hospitals on the same campus … Other features noted and recorded at the time of surgery included the rotator cuff tissue quality, the level of mobility of the tendon, and the repair quality. Each was graded using a 4-point Likert scale (fair, good, very good, or excellent).

The rotator cuff tendon edge and the footprint at the greater tuberosity were debrided with an arthroscopic shaver. With a view either from the bursal or the articular side, the torn tendon was anchored into the bone. Anchors were placed in a single row and consisted of 1 inverted mattress suture per anchor (Opus Magnum 2, ArthroCare Corps; Smith & Nephew) … Anchors were implanted using this method, the number of which was dependent on the size of the tear.

本段主要介绍所纳入病例手术的地点,以及研究所涉及的手术方法和技巧,并阐明手术中所需要记录的数据及评分。

Rehabilitation

Immediately after surgery, patients were placed in a modified sling containing a small abduction pillow (UltraSling; DJO Global), which was worn for 6 weeks. Each patient was prescribed a standardized rehabilitation program, to be completed at home. Standard postoperative analgesia included 7 days of 500 mg paracetamol 18 mg codeine every 4 hours and 5 mg oxycodone as needed … Active overhead activities were not recommended until 3 months after surgery. Patients were not permitted to lift more than 5 kg until 3 months after surgery.

本段为术后标准化康复计划的介绍,包括对术后镇痛、药物治疗及术后各阶段的活动锻炼计划的详细阐述。

Patient evaluation

Sutures were removed 1 week after surgery and patients completed a pain questionnaire during this visit. All patients were assessed for both pain and function in a similar fashion at 6, 12, and 24 weeks after surgery. A modified L'Insalata questionnaire with Likert scales was used. Questions involving the severity of pain were graded on a 5-point scale of 0 to 4, with 0 indicating mild and 4 indicating very severe pain … Patient-reported stiffness was also assessed using a 5-point scale of 0 to 4, with 0 indicating none at all and 4 indicating very stiff.

本段详细说明研究所需的术后各项评分的获取,包括问卷调查进行的具体时间段、具体的问卷类型、评分细则等。

第三部分:介绍数据的统计学分析方法。

Statistical analysis

Spearman correlation coefficient tests were performed, comparing all parameters of the study … Based on these new cutoffs, logistical regression formulas were created to predict the likelihood of a patient experiencing frequent or severe postoperative pain at 6 weeks after surgery.

本段介绍研究所采用的统计学分析方法:使用斯皮尔曼等级相关系数检验,并运用 logistic 回归来预测未来频繁或严重疼痛的可能性。

例 2

Methods

第一部分:描述数据资料的来源及样本纳入/排除标准。

Patients

Patients aged between 18 and 60 without primary neurological deficit who were treated nonoperatively for a type A thoracolumbar (T6 - L5) spinal fracture (according to the comprehensive classification) at the University Medical Centre Groningen, the Netherlands, were eligible for the study. All patients were treated between 1993 and 2000. Exclusion criteria were … Patients were sent a letter requesting their participation along with two questionnaires for completion. Medical files of all included patients were reviewed to obtain data on late onset pain and late onset neurological deficits.

首段阐述研究对象的纳入/排除标准,以及采用的相关数据。

第二部分:描述研究相关定义及观察结果指标。

Treatment

Treatment was initialized in our hospital and continued in the outpatient clinic or in a rehabilitation center. A senior staff member was responsible for deciding on the preferred method of therapy. Treatment consisted of two to six weeks bed rest (or Stryker frame). After this period, type A1.3, A2, and A3 fractures were … The brace was worn for nine months—the first six months' night and day, the last three months only during the daytime.

本段给出了研究所采用的治疗及康复计划的相关定义。

Functional outcome

Functional outcome was measured using two disease-specific questionnaires: the visual analogue scale spine score (VAS) and the Roland-Morris disability questionnaire (RMDQ). The VAS, developed for use in patients with a spinal fracture, consists of 19 items … The RMDQ measures … The RMDQ was found to be a sensitive, reliable, and valid instrument for measuring physical impairment due to back pain.

本段详细描述所采用的结果指标的具体评分标准及其含义。

第三部分:对数据进行统计学分析。

Statistical analysis

Statistical analysis was carried out using SPSS 11.0 (SPSS Inc., Chicago, Illinois). VAS and RMDQ scores four and ten years after the trauma were compared by means of the paired-sample t test. To analyze the effect of independent variables (i.e. age, gender, fracture type, and duration of time between measurements) on VAS and RMDQ difference scores (i.e. mid-term, long-term), a linear regression analysis was performed. A P value of 0.05 was considered to be of statistical significance.

本段具体说明研究分析所采用的统计学方法和软件类型。

论文研读

英文论文

Prevalence, distribution, and morphology of ossification of the ligamentum flavum: a population study of one thousand seven hundred thirty-Six magnetic resonance imaging scans

Jiongjiong Guo, Keith D. K. Luk, Jaro Karppinen, Huilin Yang, Kenneth M. C. Cheung

Abstract

Study design Large scale, cross-sectional imaging study of a general population.

Objectives To evaluate the prevalence, morphology, and distribution of ossification of the ligamentum flavum (OLF) in a population, and synthesize the scientific literature on the prevalence of OLF and some factors associated with its occurrence.

Summary of background data OLF is a rare disease in which the pathogenesis has not been conclusively established. Little is known about its epidemiology. To date, there is no study that comprehensively assessed the distribution and prevalence of OLF in the whole spine using magnetic resonance imaging (MRI).

Methods A total of 1,736 southern Chinese volunteers (1,068 women, 668 men) between 8 and 88 years of age (mean, 38 years) were recruited by open invitation. MRI was administered to all the participants. T2-weighted, 5-mm spin-echo MRI sequences of the whole spine were obtained. Presence of OLF was identified as an area of low signal intensity in the T2 sagittal sequence located in the posterior part of the spinal canal, and subsequently confirmed by computed tomography scans showing areas of ossification within the ligamentum flavum.

The distribution of OLF was classified into 3 types: the isolated type, continuous type, and noncontinuous type. While the morphology of the lesion was classified into triangular, round, and beak shapes based on the pattern of ossification on T2-weighted sagittal MRIs.

Results   OLF was identified in a total of 66 subjects or 3.8% of the population (52 women and 14 men). In 45(68.2%) cases, OLF was present at a single-level (isolated type), whereas in 21 (31.8%) cases OLF was present at multiple levels. The isolated type was found in 45 (68.2%) cases, continuous type in 11(16.7%), and noncontinuous type in 10 (15.2%). The most common site of involvement is the lower thoracic spine, but they can also occur in the upper thoracic spine. The majority of the segments had a round morphology ($n = 75$, 81.5%), while 17 (18.5%) segments were triangular in shape. A literature review of the past 26 years showed only 4 reports on the prevalence of OLF, all were in special patient groups.

Conclusions   Case reports have described postoperative paraplegia from failure to identify and decompress all stenotic segments of OLF. This study demonstrated that OLF is not uncommon, and that some 15% of the lesions are noncontinuous, and therefore could be missed. The authors recommend that for patients undergoing surgical decompression for 1 level of OLF, the whole spine should be routinely screened for other stenotic segments. Failure to do so could result in paraplegia from the nondecompressed levels.

Ossification of the ligamentum flavum (OLF), also known as ossification of the yellow ligament (OYL), has been recognized as a cause of myeloradiculopathy since it was first reported by Polgar in 1920. Like ossification of the posterior longitudinal ligament, OLF is a relatively common pathologic condition in Japan, but its prevalence has not been studied as vigorously as ossification of the posterior longitudinal ligament. Other than the Japanese, there have been some scattered case reports among whites, Africans, Arabs, and Chinese. The epidemiology and etiology of OLF remains obscure. In a review of the English literature of the past 27 years, there was only one published report of the prevalence of OLF in a Japanese population.

OLF can be shown on magnetic resonance imaging (MRI). The T2-weighted sagittal image is the sequence of choice for screening the longitudinal extent of OLF, with increased diagnostic accuracy when combined with computed tomography (CT). To date, there is no study that comprehensively examined the whole spine using MRI to assess the prevalence, distribution, and morphology of OLF. For this reason, and as part of a large ongoing study on genetics and intervertebral disc degeneration in the Southern Chinese, we conducted a prospective MRI surveillance of the whole spine. We also conducted a review and try to determine more systematically the prevalence of OLF in different ethnic population. These available data allowed us to add to our current knowledge on the prevalence of OLF.

Materials and methods

Participants

The local ethics committee approved the study, and informed consent was obtained. A cross-sectional survey was conducted from February 2001 to September 2006. Volunteers of southern Chinese origin were recruited from the population by open invitation. The exclusion criteria included pregnancy, severe osteoporosis, previous spinal surgery, treated or untreated central nervous system impairment, fracture, functional illiteracy, subjects unable to undergo MRI scanning because of ferromagnetic implants, severe claustrophobia, or inability to tolerate positioning for MRI.

Radiologic examination

Before August 2004, 991 volunteers obtained their MRI examinations from the University MRI research facility using a 0.2-T Profile open MRI system (General Electric Medical System, Milwaukee, WI). Sagittal T2-weighted fast spin-echo sequences (TR, 3,000 milliseconds; TE, 92 milliseconds; slice thickness, 5 mm) were used to image the whole spine with a built-in flexible body coil. Between August 2004 and September 2006, 745 volunteers were examined at the local hospital using a 1.5-T clinical MRI (General Electric Medical System, Milwaukee, WI). Sagittal T2-weighted fast spin-echo sequences (TR, 3,325 milliseconds; TE, 85 milliseconds; slice thickness, 5 mm) were used. All MRIs were read by 2 experienced physicians (K. M. C. C. and J. K.), differences were settled by consensus. After MRI documented the suspected levels, CT scans were performed to confirm the diagnosis.

OLF appears as areas of hypointense signal intensity at the level of the posterior margin of the spinal canal in T2-weighted images, compromising the spinal canal, and causing spinal cord compression. On CT scans, the lesions are seen as ossified masses arising from the lamina or facet joints (Figure 1).

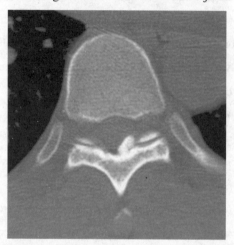

Figure 1 Axial CT of OLF. Ossified lesion is connected and arising from the lamina

The OLF were further classified by patterns of involvement as the isolated type (lesion involving 1 lamina); the continuous type (continuous lesion along 2 or more laminae); and the noncontinuous type (isolated or continuous at intervals). Morphologically the lesions were classified into triangular, round, or beak types based on the pattern of ossification visualized on T2-weighted sagittal MRIs. Because ossification types may be different on each sagittal MRI cuts, the cut that shows the OLF to be the largest was chosen for the purpose of the classification.

Results

Description of study participants and radiologic findings

A total of 1,736 participants were recruited, there were 1,068 women and 668 men. Informed consent was obtained. Subjects were told that they were volunteering for a study of genetic factors in intervertebral disc degeneration. The mean age was 38 years (range, 8 – 88 years). About 1,679 subjects were younger than 55 years of age. OLF was identified in 52 women and 14 men. Their mean age was 46 years (range, 30 – 65 years). The distribution of OLF by age and gender is shown in Table 1. In 45 cases (68.2%), OLF was present only at a single-level, whereas in 21cases (31.8%) OLF was present at multiple levels. Of the later group, OLF was present at 2 levels in 17 cases, at 3 levels in 3 cases, at 4 levels in 1 case. There were 92 OLF segments in total and a clear geographic grouping in its distribution: 48 segments (52.2%) were located in the lower thoracic spine (T9 – T12), 24 (26.1%) in the upper thoracic spine (T1 – T4), and only 15 (16.3%) in the mid-thoracic spine (T5 – T8). Four (4.3%) were in the cervical spine and 1 (0.1%) in the lumbar spine. The 3 most commonly affected levels were T10 – T11, T9 – T10, and T3 – T4 (Figure 2).

Table 1　Numbers and percent of OLF by age and gender (N, %)

Age groups	N	OLF		
		Male	Female	Total
Age≤25	287	0	0	0
25 < Age≤35	406	0	2(0.84%)	2(0.49%)
35 < Age≤45	493	6(3.41%)	18(5.68%)	24(4.87%)
Age >45	550	8(3.86%)	32(9.33%)	40(7.27%)
Total	1736	14(2.10%)	52(4.87%)	66(3.80%)

OLF indicates ossification of the ligamentum flavum.

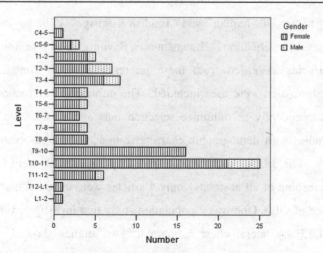

Figure 2　Distribution of OLF sites between genders

Three patterns of involvement were evident. The isolated type occurred in 45 cases（68.2%）; the continuous type occurred in 11 cases（16.7%）; and the noncontinuous type occurred in 10 cases（15.2%）. Morphologically, among the 92 ossification segments, 17（18.5%）were triangular type, 75（81.5%）were round type（Figure 3 A – C）.

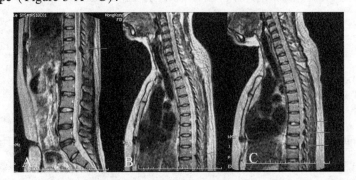

Figure 3   T2-weighted sagittal MRIs of examples of types of OLF by site and morphology; A isolated, B non-continuous, round（upper）, triangular（lower）, C continuous. A, an OLF lesion involving T11/12 lamina（arrow）; B, two isolated OLF lesions at T2/3 and T10/11 lamina（arrow）, morphologically the upper lesion was classified as a round type and the lower lesion was classified as a triangular type; C, a continuous OLF lesion of three levels from T7 to T10（arrow）

Literature review process and results

An English literature search was conducted on Ovid MEDLINE covering the span from 1980 to 2006 to identify reports of OLF. The search was performed with limiting factors of "human" and "English language". The key words for the search included ossification, ligamentum flavum, and yellow ligament. Additional articles identified from these references, which contained relevant supporting information were then included. The information extraction of articles was done independently to minimize selection bias and errors. We focused on reviewing studies with demographic characterization, radiologic examination and epidemiology. The articles without a clear description of OLF were excluded.

After screening of all abstracts, only 4 articles were included that reported on the prevalence of OLF. One was a population study that investigated the incidence of thoracic OLF by lateral chest radiograph. Two studies showed incidence of lumbar OLF by CT or lumbosacral radiographs in the sample extracted from the authors' hospital patients. One study reported 26 cases of OLF in 100 patients through chest and abdominal CT. The results of the studies are summarized in Table 2. Two studies published in French and Japanese were also summarized.

Table 2   Reported prevalence of OLF

Author	Country	Year	Sample size	Target sample	Age (yr)	Radiologic methods	OLF levels	Prevalence	Deficiency of the study
Kudo et al.	Japan	1983	1 744	Normal population	20 – 40	Lateral chest radiographs	Mainly from T9 to L1	6.2% ,in men 4.8% in women	Thoracic OLF and results may be underestimated by radiographs
Williams	USA	1984	100	Patients	5 – 89	CT of chest and abdominal	Thoracic and lumbar spine	26%	White patients sample
Kurihara et al.	Japan	1988	2 403	Patients	25 – 85	Lumbosacral roentgenogram	24.7% at L2 –L3, 22.5% at L1 –L2, and 1.9% in L3 –L4	8.6%	Lumbar OLF, patients sample, and results may be underestimated
Al-Orainy and Kolawole	Saudi Arabia	1998	82	Patients	1 – 70	CT of the lumbar spine	Lumbar	35.4%	Lumbar OLF, patients sample

OLF indicates ossification of the ligamentum flavum.

Discussion

This study was made possible because it was a part of a large scale genetic study on intervertebral disc degeneration. Our genetic study has already demonstrated, by microsatellite marker analysis, that this volunteer population is representative of the Southern Chinese population. The whole spine MRIs made it easier to diagnose OLF in early stages. Thus we believe that this is the largest population based study to date with accurate diagnosis using MRIs for screening, and CT scans for verification.

Till now, insufficient epidemiological data limited our knowledge. OLF is usually asymptomatic when lesions are small. This is supported by the present study. In Japan, it has been reported that 25% of thoracic OLF are asymptomatic. Although OLF has been considered uncommon among whites, 1

American and 1 Belgian study estimated the prevalence of OLF to be 26% and 5.44%, respectively. The incidence among the African American population seems to be low, with only 4 cases reported in the literature. However, all these studies are limited by their sample size, region of the spine imaged, or the method of diagnosis. Our population study suggests that the overall prevalence within the Southern Chinese population is 3.8%.

It is difficult to compare the present results with others directly because of differences in methods of diagnosis and that our subjects had no neurologic complaints (Table 2). Age could be a factor related to symptoms and our OLF cases were relatively young.

The ossification may grow in the coming years thereby occupying the rest of the spinal canal and resulting in symptoms of spinal cord compression. Long-term longitudinal follow-up will be needed to see whether this is the case. The mean age of most previously reported series ranged from 50 to 60 years and most presented with neurology requiring surgery. There was only one population study that used lateral thoracic radiographs and occasionally tomograms for diagnosis of OLF. In that study, the prevalence of OLF in men was the highest (12.1%) in the elderly population (>80 years) while the highest rate (10.7%) in women occurred in a 40 – 49-year-old group. However, plain radiographs are not a sensitive method of diagnosis as the radiopaque shadow representing OLF can be obscured by superimposed bony structures. CT scan is still the standard for the documentation of OLF as it can clearly identify the areas of ossification.

Our data show that the presence of OLF is age dependent, with the prevalence rising from 0.5% under 35 years of age to 5% between 35 and 45 years, and 7% over 45 years of age. This is not too surprising and would be in accordance with our clinical experience, in that symptomatic OLF tends to be present among those over 50 years of age. Interestingly, the present study demonstrated a higher prevalence rate in women (5%) than men (2%). A male preponderance was reported in most previous series, although in 2 studies a higher rate of OLF was found in female patients.

OLF most frequently occurred in the lower-thoracic region (T10 – T12).

This may be because this region is transitioning from the thoracic to the lumbar spine, where there is less anatomic protection from the rib cage. Thus, it is more prone to degeneration due to the high tensile forces present in the posterior column. As a result, collagen hyperplasia and hypertrophy may occur, with subsequent deposition of calcium pyrophosphate dehydrate and calcium hydroxyapatite in the ligament, resulting in OLF. Alternatively, it has also been suggested that OLF is a degenerative response to the microinjury of the ligamentum flavum.

The second most common location in this study was the upper thoracic spine (T1 – T4). While our subjects were asymptomatic, it has been suggested that these cases are more likely to be symptomatic since the thoracic kyphosis would result in stretching of the spinal cord over the lesion. Moreover, this is the part of the spinal cord with the poorest collateral circulation.

OLF is thought to have a different etiology to calcification of the ligamentum flavum (LF). Ossification involves the lamina while calcification does not (Figure 4). This distinction may be of significance in relation to their etiology. All cases described in the current study involved the lamina and are true ossification. However, regardless of whether the lesion is calcified, ossified, or even a spinal tumor, they are all shown as the presence of low signal intensity mass in the posterior aspect of the spinal canal on T1, T2, and proton density weighted MRI images. On the issue of how to differentiate facet osteophytes with OLF, sometimes ossification or calcification of the facet capsule can be mistaken as OLF. The ossification process started at the base of the ligament with endochondral ossification of the hypertrophied fibrous tissue. Early ossification, in linear form, usually was found on the medial capsular side of the ligament, and then grew into the canal. However, facet osteophytes were usually detected on the lateral side of the joint with severer degenerations. There is sometimes a gap between the OLF and facet surface. OLF has graduation of the ossification by CT, also in some cases. A clear differential diagnosis of these diseases can only be made on CT scans.

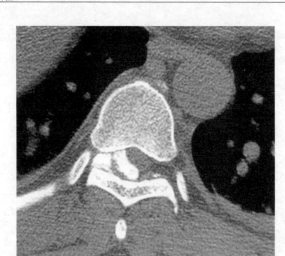

Figure 4 **Axial CT of calcification of ligamentum flavum. Calcification of the ligamentum flavum on axial CT showed that the calcified mass is separate and does not involve the bony lamina**

A number of authors have suggested that a whole spine T2-weighted sagittal MRI should be performed for all OLF patients, as there is a chance of multiple level lesion and combined pathologies such as hidden cervical and lumbar stenosis. Our study would suggest that almost 1/3 (32%) have more than one level of the spine involved, although in the majority the lesions are still restricted to the thoracic spine, 4% are in the cervical and 0.1% in the lumbar spine. OLF was recognized by the presence of a triangular or hemispheric area of low signal intensity at the level of the posterior margin of the canal. Because the ligamentum flavum is the thinnest in the midline, OLF is usually more evident in parasagittal MRI images. In the present study, OLF was classified by 2 methods on MRI. One is according to the geographic distribution and the other is according to the morphology of the ossification. Most ossification segments in the present study were of a round type (81.5%). We did not find any beak type within our population. This may be because beak types are uncommon within our population, or that beak types tend to present early with neurologic deficit, and are therefore not seen in an asymptomatic population study. The clinical significance of these different forms of OLF will require further study.

Importantly, our study identified that multiple lesions can occur in 32% of cases, and that 15% of which are noncontinuous in nature. Missed multiple level lesions can have serious consequences. There have been reports of thoracic paraplegia developing after lumbar decompressive surgery due to stenosis and spinal cord compression from missed OLF in the thoracic spine.

Conclusions

This is the first large scale population study of OLF in the Chinese population. It reported an overall prevalence of OLF to be 3.8%. However, the prevalence is age-dependent and that it is commoner in females. About 32% of the subjects have multiple level lesions, with 15% being noncontinuous in nature.

SPINE. 2010;35(1):151－156

DOI:10.1097/BRS obo13e318/b3f779

词　汇

ossification	*n.* 骨化;成骨;(思想的)僵化
prevalence	*n.* 患病率;流行;普遍
epidemiology	*n.* 流行病学;传染病学
thoracic	*adj.* [解剖]胸的;[解剖]胸廓的
ligament	*n.* 韧带;纽带,系带
ethics	*n.* 伦理学;伦理观;道德标准
illiteracy	*n.* 文盲;无知
segment	*n.* 段,部分;(水果或花的)瓣;(动物的)节;弓形
abdominal	*adj.* 腹部的;有腹鳍的

译　文

黄韧带骨化的患病率、分布和形态:1 736 例磁共振成像人群研究

摘要

设计　对普通人群的一项大规模的横断面影像研究。

目的　了解黄韧带骨化(OLF)在人群中的患病率、形态和分布,综述有关 OLF 患病率及其相关因素的文献。

背景资料　OLF 是一种罕见的疾病,其发病机制尚未明确。人们对其流行病学知之甚少。到目前为止,还没有使用磁共振成像(MRI)全面评估 OLF

在全脊柱中的分布和患病率的研究。

方法 我们公开招募了 1 736 名地区的志愿者,其中女性 1 068 人、男性 668 人,年龄为8—88岁,平均年龄为 38 岁。所有参与者均接受 MRI 检查。我们得到全脊柱下 T$_2$ 加权 5 毫米自旋回波 MRI 序列。OLF 被确认为存在于椎管后部的 T2 矢状位序列中的低信号区域,随后这一点通过计算机断层扫描显示黄韧带内的骨化区而得到证实。OLF 的分布可分为三种类型:孤立型、连续型和非连续型。根据 T2 加权矢状位 MRI 上的骨化类型,病变的形态可分为三角形、圆形和喙状。

结果 共 66 例受试者(女性 52 例,男性 14 例)被诊断为黄韧带骨化,占总人数的 3.8%。单节段(孤立型)为 45 例(68.2%),多节段为 21 例(31.8%)。其中孤立型为 45 例(68.2%),连续型为 11 例(16.7%),非连续型为 10 例(15.2%)。最常见的受累部位是下胸椎,但也发生在上胸椎。大多数节段形态为圆形($n = 75$, 81.5%),17 个节段(18.5%)呈三角形。根据过去 26 年的文献回顾,仅有 4 份关于 OLF 患病率的报告,均为特殊患者。

结论 病例报告描述了所有由于未能诊断和对 OLF 所有狭窄节段减压而导致的术后截瘫病例。这项研究表明,OLF 并不少见,大约 15% 的病变是不连续的,因此可能会被漏诊。作者建议,接受单节段 OLF 手术减压治疗的患者应接受常规的整个脊柱其他狭窄节段的筛查。如果做不到这一点,可能会导致非减压水平的截瘫。

黄韧带骨化(OLF),又称 OYL,自 1920 年 Polgar 首次对其进行报告以来,一直被认为是引起脊髓小管病变的原因之一。与后纵韧带骨化一样,在日本 OLF 是一种相对常见的病理状态,但其患病率并没有像后纵韧带骨化那样得到广泛的研究。除日本人外,在白人、非洲人、阿拉伯人和中国人中也有一些零散的病例报告。OLF 的流行病学和病因尚不清楚。回顾过去 27 年的文献,已发表的只有一篇关于日本人群中 OLF 患病率的报告。

磁共振成像(MRI)可显示 OLF。T2 加权矢状位图像是筛查 OLF 纵向范围的首选序列,结合 CT 可提高诊断准确率。迄今为止,还没有研究通过 MRI 对全脊柱进行全面检查来评估 OLF 的患病率、分布和形态。出于这个原因,作为正在进行的关于中国南方人遗传学和椎间盘退变的大型研究的一部分,我们对整个脊柱进行了前瞻性的 MRI 监测。我们还进行了回顾,试图更系统地确定 OLF 在不同种族人群中的患病率。这些数据能够增加我们目前对 OLF 患病率的了解。

材料与方法

研究对象

当地伦理委员会批准了这项研究，并且我们获得了知情同意。2001 年 2 月至 2006 年 9 月，我们进行了一项横断面调查。我们公开招募了华南地区的志愿者。排除标准包括怀孕、严重骨质疏松症、既往脊柱手术、中枢神经系统损伤治疗或未治疗、骨折、功能性文盲、因磁性金属植入物而无法接受 MRI 扫描、严重幽闭恐惧症或无法耐受 MRI 定位。

放射检查

2004 年 8 月之前，991 名志愿者使用大学 MRI 研究设施进行 MRI 检查（威斯康星州密尔沃基通用电气医疗系统），使用矢状位 T2 加权快速自旋回波序列（TR，3 000 毫秒；TE，92 毫秒；层厚，5 厘米），用内置柔性线圈对全脊柱进行成像。2004 年 8 月至 2006 年 9 月，745 名志愿者在当地医院接受了 1.5-T 临床 MRI（威斯康星州密尔沃基通用电气医疗系统）的检查，使用矢状位 T2 加权快速自旋回波序列（TR，3 325 毫秒；TE，85 毫秒；层厚，5 厘米）。所有的 MRI 均由 2 名经验丰富的医生阅片，并协商一致。在 MRI 描记了可疑水平后，医生进行 CT 扫描以确诊。

OLF 在 T2 加权矢位图像上表现为椎管后缘水平的低信号区域，损害椎管，并导致脊髓受压。在 CT 扫描上，病变表现为椎板或小关节的骨化性肿块（图 1）。

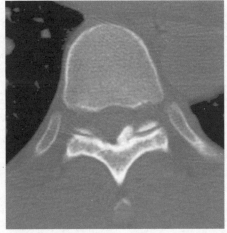

图 1 OLF 的 CT 轴位，骨化病变发自椎板

OLF 按受累类型进一步分为孤立型(累及 1 个椎板)、连续型(沿 2 个或 2 个以上椎板连续)和非连续型(孤立或间隔连续)。根据 T2 加权矢状位 MRI 上显示的骨化模式,病变在形态上分为三角形、圆形或喙状。每个矢状面 MRI 切面上的骨化类型可能不同,因此选择显示 OLF 最大的切面进行分类。

结果

研究对象和放射学发现

研究总共招募了 1 736 名研究对象,其中女性 1 068 名、男性 668 名。研究均获得研究对象知情同意。受试者被告知,他们是自愿参加椎间盘退变遗传因素研究的。研究对象的平均年龄为 38 岁(区间为 8—88 岁),其中约有 1 679 名受试者的年龄在 55 岁以下。我们在 52 名女性和 14 名男性中发现了 OLF,平均年龄为 46 岁(区间为 30—65 岁)。OLF 的年龄和性别分布见表 1。45 例(68.2%)中 OLF 仅存在于单个节段,而 21 例(31.8%)中 OLF 存在于多个节段。后者中,OLF 存在于 2 个节段的为 17 例,存在于 3 个节段的为 3 例,存在于 4 个节段的为 1 例。OLF 共 92 个节段,位置分型清楚:下胸椎(T9—T12)48 个节段(52.2%),上胸椎(T1—T4)24 个节段(26.1%),中胸椎(T5—T8)15 个节段(16.3%)。其中,颈椎有 4 例(4.3%),腰椎有 1 例(0.1%)。受影响最大的 3 个水平是 T10—T11、T9—T10 和 T3—T4(图 2)。

表 1 按年龄和性别划分的 OLF 数量和百分比(数值,%)

年龄分组	数量	OLF		
		男性	女性	总数
年龄≤25	287	0	0	0
25 < 年龄≤35	406	0	2(0.84%)	2(0.49%)
35 < 年龄≤45	493	6(3.41%)	18(5.68%)	24(4.87%)
年龄 > 45	550	8(3.86%)	32(9.33%)	40(7.27%)
总数	1 736	14(2.10%)	52(4.87%)	66(3.80%)

OLF 表示黄韧带骨化。

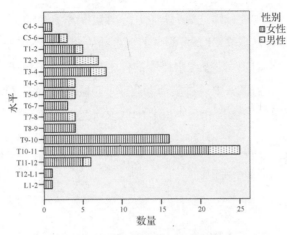

图 2 OLF 在不同性别之间的分布

OLF 分为 3 型:孤立型,45 例(68.2%);连续型,11 例(16.7%);非连续型,10 例(15.2%)。形态上,92 个骨化节段中,三角形为 17 个(18.5%),圆形为 75 个(81.5%)(图 3)。

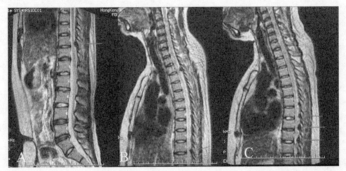

图 3 T2 加权矢状位 MRI 按部位和形态分型:A 孤立,B 不连续,圆形(上),三角形(下),C 连续。A 为累及 T11/12 椎板的 OLF 病灶(箭头);B 为 T2/3 和 T10/11 椎板的孤立性 OLF 病变(箭头),形态上病变上部为圆形,下部为三角形;C 为从 T7 到 T10 连续三个节段的 OLF 病变(箭头)

文献综述与结果

我们用 Ovid MEDLINE 数据库进行文献检索,时间跨度为 1980—2006 年,来检索 OLF 的报告文献。检索有"人"和"英语"的限制。检索的关键词包括"骨化""黄韧带""黄色韧带"。从这些参考文献中确定的包含相关支持信息的其他文章随后也被包括在内。文章的信息提取是独立进行的,这样可以最大限度地减少选择偏差和错误。我们重点回顾了人口特征、放射学检查和流行病学方面的研究,排除未明确描述 OLF 的文章。

对所有文献摘要进行筛选后,只有 4 篇文献报告了 OLF 的患病率。一篇是通过侧位胸片研究胸段 OLF 发病率的人群研究。两项研究是通过 CT 或腰骶 X 线片,在从作者的医院患者中提取的样本中显示腰椎 OLF 的发病率。一项研究报告了 100 例患者中通过胸部和腹部 CT 检查的 26 例 OLF。研究结果见表 2。我们还总结了法国和日本发表的两项研究。

表 2　报告的 OLF 患病率

作者	国家	年份/年	样本量	目标样本	年龄/岁	放射方法	OLF水平	发生率	研究缺陷
Kudo 等	日本	1983	1 744	普通人群	20—40	侧位胸片	主要来自 T9 – L1	男6.2%,女4.8%	X 线片可能低估胸部 OLF 和结果
Williams	美国	1984	100	患者	5—89	胸腹部 CT	胸腰椎	26%	白人患者样本
Kurihara 等	日本	1988	2 403	患者	25—85	腰骶X 线	24.7% L2 – L3, 22.5% L1 – L2, 1.9% L3 – L4	8.6%	腰椎 OLF、患者样本和结果可能被低估
Al-Orainy 和 Kolawole	沙特阿拉伯	1998	82	患者	1—70	腰椎 CT	腰椎	35.4%	腰椎 OLF,患者样本

OLF 表示黄韧带骨化。

讨论

这项研究得益于本身是一项关于椎间盘退变的大规模遗传学研究的一部分。我们的遗传学研究已经证明,这个志愿者群体是华南地区人群的代表。全脊椎磁共振成像使 OLF 的早期诊断变得更容易,因此我们相信这是迄今为止最大的基于人群的研究,研究使用 MRI 进行筛查,通过 CT 扫描进行验证,从而做出准确的诊断。

到目前为止,流行病学数据不足限制了我们的认知。当病灶很小时,OLF通常是无症状的,这一点得到了本研究的支持。在日本,有报告称 25% 的胸段 OLF 是无症状的。虽然 OLF 在白人中很少见,但 1 项美国研究和 1 项比利时研究估计 OLF 的患病率分别为 26% 和 5.44%。非洲裔美国人的发病率似乎很低,文献报告中只有4例。但所有这些研究都受到样本量、脊柱成像区域或诊断方法的限制。我们的人口研究表明,华南地区人口的总体患病率为3.8%。

因为诊断方法不同,我们很难将目前的结果与其他结果直接比较,而且我们的受试者没有神经学方面的主诉(表2)。年龄可能是一个与症状相关的因素,我们的OLF病例相对年轻。

骨化可能会在接下来的几年里扩大,从而占据椎管的其余部分,导致出现脊髓受压症状。验证是否会如此需要长期的纵向随访。以前报告的大多数患者的平均年龄从50岁到60岁不等,大多数人表现为需要手术的神经疾病。只有一项人群研究使用侧位胸片和少数的体层摄片来诊断OLF。在该研究中,男性的OLF患病率在老年人群(>80岁)中最高(12.1%),而女性的最高患病率(10.7%)是发生在40—49岁年龄组。然而,X线平片并不是一种敏感的诊断方法,因为代表OLF的不透射线的阴影可能会被叠加的骨性结构所掩盖,CT扫描仍然是OLF的诊断标准,因为可以清楚地识别骨化区。

我们的数据显示,OLF的存在与年龄有关,患病率从35岁以下的0.5%上升到35—45岁的5%,以及45岁以上的7%。这并不令人惊讶,与我们的临床经验是一致的,有症状的OLF往往出现在50岁以上的人群中。有趣的是,本研究显示女性的患病率(5%)高于男性的患病率(2%)。尽管两项研究发现女性患者中OLF的发生率较高,但在大多数以前的系列报告中,男性患者是更高的。

OLF多见于下胸椎(T10—T12)。这可能是因为这一区域是胸椎到腰椎的过渡区,此部位对肋骨的解剖学保护较少。由于后柱存在的高张力,此部位更容易退化。因此,胶原增生和肥大可能会发生,继而韧带中沉积焦磷酸钙和羟基磷灰石,导致出现OLF。另外,也有人认为OLF是对黄韧带微损伤的退行性反应。

本研究中第二个最常见的部位是上胸椎(T1—T4)。虽然我们的研究对象没有症状,但有人认为这些病例更有可能出现症状,因为胸椎后凸会导致脊髓病变延伸,而且这是侧支循环最差的部分。

OLF被认为与黄韧带钙化(LF)有不同的病因。骨化累及椎板,而钙化不累及椎板(图4),这种区别可能与其病因有关。目前研究中描述的所有病例均累及椎板,为真正的骨化。然而,无论病变是钙化、骨化,还是脊椎肿瘤,在

T1、T2 和质子密度加权 MRI 图像上均表现为椎管后方的低信号肿块。如何鉴别小关节骨赘与 OLF 是一个问题,有时医生会将小关节囊骨化或钙化误诊为 OLF。骨化过程始于韧带底部,肥大的纤维组织软骨内骨化,早期骨化呈线形,多见于韧带的内侧包膜,然后长入管内。但关节外侧常可见小关节骨赘,退变程度较重。OLF 和小平面之间有时会有间隙。OLF 在 CT 上有骨化分级,部分病例也有骨化。只有通过 CT 扫描才能对这些疾病做出明确的鉴别诊断。

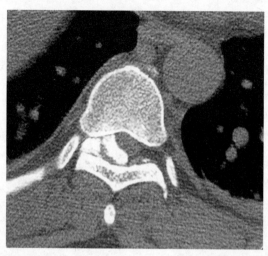

图 4 黄韧带钙化的轴位 CT 表现。轴位 CT 上黄韧带钙化显示钙化肿块是分离的,不累及骨板

一些作者建议对所有 OLF 患者进行全脊柱 T2 加权矢状位 MRI 检查,原因是有可能出现多个节段的病变,以及隐匿性颈椎和腰椎狭窄等合并病变。我们的研究表明,近 1/3(32%)的患者有多个水平的脊柱受累,大多数病变仍然局限于胸椎,4% 位于颈椎,0.1% 位于腰椎。OLF 是由椎管后缘水平的三角形或半球低信号区识别的,由于黄韧带位于中线最薄处,OLF 通常在矢状面附近的 MRI 图像上更明显。本研究在 MRI 上用两种方法对 OLF 进行了分类。一种是根据位置分布,另一种是根据骨化的形态。骨化节段多为圆形(81.5%)。我们在研究人群中没有被发现任何喙状。这可能是因为喙状在我们的人群中并不常见,或者喙状较早出现神经功能障碍,因此在无症状的人群研究中没有被发现。OLF 分型的临床意义还需要进一步的研究。

重要的是我们的研究发现,32% 的病例可以发生多处病变,15% 的病例是不连续的。漏诊的多节段病变可能会造成严重后果。有报告称,腰椎减压术后由于遗漏胸椎的 OLF 造成的狭窄和脊髓受压,可能导致截瘫。

结论

这是首次在中国人口中进行的大规模 OLF 人群研究。据报告,OLF 的总体患病率为 3.8%。然而,患病率与年龄有关,而且在女性中更为常见。大约 32% 的受试者有多个节段的病变,其中实际上 15% 是不连续的。

第七章

结果的撰写

结果(results)部分是一篇医学论文的绝对核心内容,是论文对主要研究成果的集中展示,也是结论的依据和数据的支撑。结果上承材料与方法部分,是由其得出的必然结果,下启讨论部分,是作者得出主要结论并形成观点与主题的基础。因此,参考论文的实验方法的读者,都会同时参考其结果部分,来对自己即将开展的相关研究进行结果预测。同样,关注结论的读者也会参考结果部分,从而对论文的学术价值做出判断。

7.1　结果的内容

结果部分主要表述材料与方法部分所述主要实验得出的主要结果,同时还应对研究对象的基本人口特征与临床特征的分布及其在各分组的比较予以详细描述。这部分主要回答该研究取得哪些成果,是论文写作从实践上升到理论层面的桥梁。

7.2　结果的撰写要点

结果部分的撰写是客观地讲述实验结果,一般不进行讨论和解释,不能简单地将实验数据和观察指标进行堆砌,更不能将一般数据不断重复,而是要重点突出、高度概括和精练。撰写时应注意以下几点:

① 列出最具代表性的数据,而不是将原始数据不加筛选地列出。对实验数据的评论应该集中在讨论部分。

② 为使论文更具整体感,结果部分可适当概述引言或者材料与方法部分。

③ 本部分的基本时态通常是一般过去时,但描述计算结果等用现在时。

④ 结果的表述一般采用文字与图、表相结合的形式,若结果数据量小,仅用文字表述便可;若结果数据量较大,采用图、表形式更能完整表达,可结合文字部分表述数据的趋势与特点。鉴于图、表的重要性,第八章会单独对图、表的撰写进行详细介绍。

⑤ 文字表述应精简,避免使用冗长的句式陈述结果或图、表。

⑥ 对结果的统计学意义进行表述时,最好避免使用 highly 之类的程度副词修饰 significant 之类的形容词。

示例

例1

Results

Overall, 73,284 patients underwent surgery for hip fracture repair between 1 October 2007 and 30 September 2011 and had information on the type of anesthesia received. Of those, 61,554 (84.0%) received general anesthesia, 6,939 (9.5%) received regional anesthesia, and 4,791 (6.5%) received both general and regional anesthesia … In total, 1,621 (2.2%) deaths occurred during hospital admission, which is consistent with previously reported findings.

首段对研究对象进行简单描述,说明纳入的总病例数、不同麻醉类型的数量及占比,以及住院期间的总死亡数量。

Baseline characteristics were generally similar across anesthetic groups, with a few differences noted. Compared with patients receiving other types of anesthesia, those receiving general anesthesia were younger, less likely to be women … Conversely, patients receiving regional anesthesia were older, more likely to be women, more likely to be admitted through the emergency department, less likely to have white or black ethnicity, and less likely to have chronic renal disease.

第二段说明接受不同类型的麻醉的病人的特征大致相似,但也具有一定的差异性:接受全麻的病人可能更年轻,是女性的可能性更小……而接受局部麻醉的病人可能年龄较大,更可能是女性或急诊入院,是黑人或白人,以及患慢性肾病的可能性较小。

Overall, 1,362(2.2%)in-hospital deaths occurred in patients receiving general anesthesia, 144(2.1%)in patients receiving regional anesthesia, and 115(2.4%)in patients receiving combined anesthesia...Similarly, in the multivariable analysis there was no statistically significant difference in mortality risk associated with the use of either regional compared with general anesthesia(0.93, 0.78 to 1.11)or combined compared with general anesthesia(1.00, 0.82 to 1.22).

第三段具体描述各种麻醉类型的死亡风险,发现各种麻醉类型的死亡风险无明显统计学差异。

The mixed effects analysis, which accounted for differences between hospitals, produced results consistent with those of the main analysis(regional v. general anesthesia 0.91, 0.75 to 1.10, and combined v. general anesthesia 0.98, 0.79 to 1.21). When the study population was extended to include those patients who had surgery on the first day of hospital admission, the results remained consistent(regional v. general anesthesia 0.91, 0.77 to 1.08, and combined v. general anesthesia 0.97, 0.82 to 1.17). Similarly, restricting the study population to patients with no diagnosis of cancer at discharge or to patients 75 years and older yielded a similar effect for regional or combined anesthesia compared with general anesthesia.

末段做进一步的统计分析,研究不同医院之间的差异:对将研究人群扩大或做进一步限制后的结果进行分析,发现各种麻醉类型的死亡风险仍无统计学意义。

例2

Results

Between October 2009 and April 2013, we assessed 1,969 patients with grade 1 or 2 ankle sprains for eligibility. Of these, 504 patients met our inclusion criteria, provided consent, and were randomised to the physiotherapy($n=254$)or the usual care($n=250$)arms of our study. One patient in the physiotherapy arm withdrew consent after randomisation and was excluded from the analysis...Given the actual observed sample size and the rates of contamination and loss to follow-up, the power to detect a 15% improvement in our primary outcome was 78% for the intent to treat analyses and 82% for our per protocol analyses.

首段承接方法部分,再次概述了材料与方法部分的内容,交代纳入/排除流程及人群相关特征。

Table 2 (intent to treat analysis) and Table 3 (per protocol analysis) show comparisons of the study arms for the primary outcome, FAOS ≥450 at three months, and the secondary outcomes of excellent FAOS at one and six months. The per protocol analysis excluded 69 participants in the physiotherapy arm who did not attend at least one protocol physiotherapy session in the first three months, as well as 26 participants in the control arm who received physiotherapy during the first three months. Neither analysis identified strong, consistent, or significant differences in primary or secondary FAOS outcomes by study arm.

Figure 3 (intent to treat analysis) and Figure 4 (per protocol analysis) show the change from baseline in total and domain specific continuous FAOS. Differences between groups in the mean change were not significant at any follow-up time point for any FAOS domain. Tables 4 and 5 show the results of the subgroup analysis. Although these indicate a benefit for physiotherapy at three months in the subgroup of patients aged <30, with a borderline significant ($P = 0.05$) interaction between treatment and age at the three-month assessment, this trend was not present at other time points and would not remain significant after any reasonable adjustment for multiple testing … In the six-month follow-up period, 19/254 (7.5%) participants in the physiotherapy arm and 21/250 (8.4%) in the usual care arm reported a re-injury of the same ankle, with no significant difference between the two trial arms ($P = 0.71$).

剩下的部分则是结合图、表,对分组后数据的结果进行比较及统计学分析:理疗组与常规护理组在恢复良好率上无明显统计学差异。

论文研读

经典文献链接:https://doi.org/10.1016/j.cell.2020.05.008

标题:Nurturing undergraduate researchers in biomedical sciences

词　汇

mentor　　　　*n.* 导师

hierarchical　　*adj.* 按等级划分的,等级制度的

novice　　　　*n.* 新手,初学者

affiliation　　　*n.* 隶属,所属单位

seminar　　　　*n.* 研讨会

symposium　　*n.* 研讨会

评　析

本文是一篇评述。评述一般是针对发表于同期期刊的论文发表评论,讨论对期刊读者或社会很重要的内容或与最近发展相关的其他主题,往往包含一些非科学主题的评论,如健康政策、经济、法律或伦理,或者本文所关注的教育。大多数期刊的评述文章为邀约撰写,不过有的主编也会考虑接受投稿。评述文章不需要遵循摘要、背景、方法、结果、结论的写作结构,只需清晰、明确地陈述出写作者的观点。

尽管不需要遵循严格的格式,但评述类论文的撰写也存在一定的要求。标题要简短,能引起读者的兴趣,如例文中 6 个词汇就表明了文章的主题"生物科学领域的本科生培养",而本科生的科研教育又是一贯被忽视的,这样新奇的角度也能激发读者的兴趣,引人注意。清晰表明观点是另一个需要重视的方面,这也是本文的亮点之一。阐述观点有多种方式,本文采用的是使用小标题的方式,简明扼要地概括每一部分的主旨,并且使每部分之间存在一定的逻辑顺序。文章首先点题,总起 fostering the next generation,讲明研究背景的同时也表明了这篇文章的意义:多数学者都是从本科阶段开始研究生涯,但目前的科研教育都集中在更高年级的学生身上,还没有系统的本科生科研培养体系。如果能够在本科阶段做好科研教育,这对学生的专业进步和发展都是

大有裨益的。接下来文章就从本科生的定位"Junior Colleges，not Laborers"、课题的开始到结束"Clarify Research Rationales and Key Methodologies，Get a Broad Perspective from the Literature，Foster Effective Scientific Communication，Solid Research Skills，Acquire Technical Expertise，Learn to Design and Manage Projects"、导师们的责任"Training for Novice Mentors"和社会应该"Call for More Opportunities"方面进行了详细的论述，从多个角度对本科生培养的必要性和具体实施方案提出了建议。

其中，给本科生的建议包括以下几点：

① 了解自己的实验的背景和方法；

② 向自己的导师提问，直至所有的疑虑都得到解答；

③ 耐心地多次练习实验技术，直到完全掌握；

④ 学习如何开展一个课题研究；

⑤ 锻炼交流能力，在公众面前展示自己的成果；

⑥ 通过阅读文献和参加学术会议拓宽自己的专业视野。

图、表的撰写

在进行医学英文论文写作时，特别是当数据量较大时，写作者要学会充分利用图(figure)和表(table)简化文字的叙述，这有利于数据的归纳、总结和比较，也可以节省版面。图和表往往能较为清楚地展示出论文的结果，是论文结果呈现最重要的一部分。它能让读者一目了然，从而使读者对研究结果产生较为直观的印象，让读者通读起来更为顺畅。

8.1 图、表的内容

（1）图

在医学英文论文中，图包括统计图和非统计图。非统计图包括影像学图片、组织学图片、解剖图片等，有些只需在图片边上添加图题即可，有些若要在论文里起到示意作用，则还须附上图注加以解释说明。在论文中使用图可以显示事物的变化趋势、联系、分布等，但对于资料的描述相对来说不够详细。

一个完整的统计图则需要包括以下几个方面：

一是图序和图题。图序和图题一般位于图的下方。图序表明图的次序。图题要简洁、清楚地描述统计图的内容。

二是纵横坐标。纵横坐标上要标明刻度。

三是标目及计量单位符号。不管是纵坐标还是横坐标，标目要居中放置，其后使用"/"，后附计量单位符号。

四是图例。图例分别说明统计图中显示的各线条、图形或颜色代表的事物,可被置于统计图的角落。

五是文字说明。如有需要,写作者可添加图注和说明,并将其置于图题下方。

(2) 表

在医学英文论文中,不同于图,表一般都是统计表。对于具体数据的详细表述,我们一般都是采用统计表的形式。使用统计表也是为了便于数据的统计学处理,所以在论文撰写中统计表的应用极为广泛。

一个完整的统计表需要包括以下几个方面:

一是横线。医学英文论文主要采用的是三线表,由顶线、底线和中间的标目线构成表的框架,两侧不需要另外的线条封口。其中,表头在顶线和标目线中间,表身在标目线和底线中间。注意,表头左上角不能用斜线,如有标目分层需要,可用短线分隔开来。

二是表序和表题。表序和表题一般位于表的上方。表序是表的次序,一篇论文往往有不止一张表格,需要标明表序来清楚区分。表题是对表格内容的概述,应简洁清晰。

三是标目。标目分为纵标目和横标目。纵标目位于表的上端,说明纵栏统计指标的具体含义;横标目位于表的左端,说明横栏各项的具体含义。

四是数据和显著性结果。表身用于填写数据和显著性结果。

五是注释。注释需要简洁明了,应位于表的底线下方。注释包括显著性结果、注脚符号或字母,以及标注的解释说明。

8.2 图、表的撰写要点

图和表是结果的重要组成部分,也是英文论文撰写的重点与难点。图和表需要结构完整、内容突出、排列规范、对比鲜明,这样才能保证读者准确理解图和表的内容。一些英文图、表的撰写注意点及常见错误或难点包括以下几个方面:

① 标题或注释要言简意赅、一目了然,不能过于烦琐。

② 结果部分插入的图、表要精确,必须符合原文内容。同时,写作者要精选图和表,体现论文写作简明的特点。

③ 对于图和表,写作者应按照其在正文出现的顺序进行编号。

④ 图的类型要与资料性质相符。

⑤ 图和表的内容要完整独立,要让读者看到图、表就理解作者想要表达的内容,不能让读者在看完图、表后还要回过头去参考正文内容来帮助理解。

⑥ 写作者应严格按照图和表的书写格式写作。图题位于底部,文字性描述位于图旁。表题位于表的上方。统计图的图例字号要比标题小 1 号。图、表的标目的首字母要大写,统计表横标目下的项目要缩进两个字母。计量单位一般采用缩写,位于统计指标或项目的后面或下面,加上括号。

⑦ 注脚可以是句子或短语,字号要小标题 1 号,可使用术语或缩写。

⑧ 国际通用的缩略词无须写全称,可直接使用;非国际通用的缩略词在正文中已有解释的也可直接使用。

示 例

例1

简单直条图

简单直条图是用相同宽度的直条的长短来表示相互独立的某统计指标值的大小。

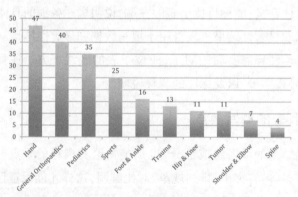

Figure 1   The most common reported primary specialist of respondents included hand, general orthopaedics, pediatric orthopaedics, and sports ($n = 209$)

例 2

堆积条形图

堆积条形图显示单个项目与整体之间的关系。堆积条形图不仅可以呈现每个系列的值,还能反映出系列的总和。

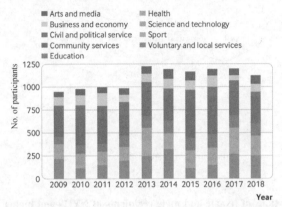

Figure 2　Distribution(%) of NYHs for each year from 2009 to 2018

例 3

饼图

饼图用于表示构成比。

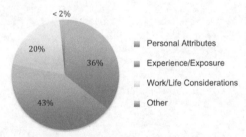

Figure 3　Potential dissuaders for women considering orthopaedic surgery represented all categories (n = 231 of 232)

例 4

线图

线图用线段的升降来表示数值的变化。

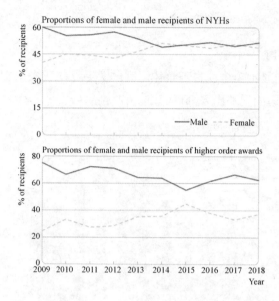

Figure 4 Proportions of female and male recipients of NYHs and higher order awards

例5

散点图

散点图用于表示两个变量或多个变量之间有无相关关系。

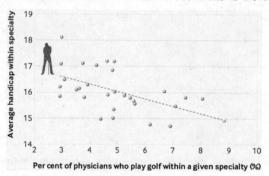

Figure 5 Relation between golf handicap and percentage of physicians who play golf, by specialty (represented by dots)

例6

箱式图

箱式图是一种可以相对直观显示一组数据分布情况的统计图。

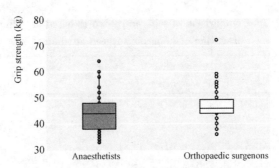

Figure 6 Box plot of grip strength（kg）by specialty

【例7】

机制图

对于比较复杂的研究方案、具有独创性的研究路径及关键步骤,我们可以借助机制图来进行辅助说明。

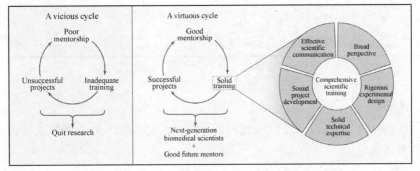

Figure 7 Fostering a virtuous cycle with good mentorship instead of a vicious style

【例8】

三线表

三线表形式简洁、功能分明、阅读方便,在英文论文写作中被推荐使用。三线表通常只有三条表线,即顶线、底线和栏目线。

Table 1 Comparision of self-control scores based on different practicing orthopaedic surgeon attributes

Variable	No. (%)	Mean ±standard deviation(range)	Median	Mean difference(95% confidence interval)	P value
Overall	655(100)	3.91 ±0.54(1.8 to 5.0)	4		
Sex				0.07(−0.05 to 0.20)	0.26
Female	82(12.5)	3.85 ±0.59(2.3 to 4.8)	3.9		
Male	573(87.5)	3.92 ±0.54(1.8 to 5.0)	4		
Varsity college sports participation				0.05(−0.03 to 0.13)	0.22
Yes	306(46.7)	3.94 ±0.54(1.8 to 5.0)	4		
No	349(53.3)	3.89 ±0.54(2.3 to 5.0)	4		
AΩA honor society status				0.02(−0.05 to 0.12)	0.40
Yes	231(35.3)	3.94 ±0.52(2.3 to 5.0)	4		
No	344(52.5)	3.93 ±0.56(1.8 to 5.0)	4		

例 9

复杂表

对多栏目、多栏数据进行表述时,简单的三线表往往无法满足表述需求,复杂表可适用。

Table 2 Baseline characteristics of study patients.

Values are numbers (percentages) unless stated otherwise

Characteristics	Full analysis set			As treated groups			
	Early ACL reconstruction (n=61)	Delayed optional ACL (n=59)	P value	Early ACL reconstruction (n=59)	Delayed ACL reconstruction (n=30)	Rehabilitation alone (n=29)	P value
Mean (SD) age (years)	26.4(5.1)	25.8(4.7)	0.47	26.5(5.1)	25.2(4.5)	26.4(4.9)	0.47
Female sex	12(20)	20(34)	0.08	12(20)	11(37)	9(31)	0.23
Mean (SD) body mass index	24.5(3.1)	23.8(2.6)	0.22	24.5(3.2)	23.3(2.0)	24.3(3.1)	0.25
Increased anteroposterior laxity	60(98) *	58(98)†	0.98	58(98) *	29(97)†	29(100)	0.61

continued

Characteristics	Full analysis set			As treated groups			
	Early ACL reconstruction (n =61)	Delayed optional ACL (n =59)	P value	Early ACL reconstruction (n =59)	Delayed ACL reconstruction (n =30)	Rehabilitation alone (n =29)	P value
Median (interquartile range) Tegner activity scale	9(7.9)	9(7.9)	0.82	9(7.9)	8.5(7.9)	9(7.9)	0.91

ACL = anterior cruciate ligament.

A comprehensive description of baseline characteristics for all included patients has been published.

*In one knee, anteroposterior laxity could not be assessed owing to pain; magnetic resonance imaging (MRI) and arthroscopy confirmed total ACL rupture.

†In one knee, anteroposterior laxity was found to be normal at baseline, but MRI and arthroscopy confirmed total ACL rupture.

论文研读

英文论文

Postoperative outcomes of tranexamic acid in patients undergoing total hip or knee arthroplasty

Abstract

Objective To determine the effectiveness and safety of perioperative tranexamic acid use in patients undergoing total hip or knee arthroplasty.

Design Retrospective cohort study; multilevel multivariable logistic regression models measured the association between tranexamic acid use in the perioperative period and outcomes.

Participants 872,416 patients who had total hip or knee arthroplasty from 2013 to 2019.

Intervention Perioperative intravenous tranexamic acid use by dose categories (none, ≤1,000 mg, 2,000 mg, and ≥3,000 mg).

Main outcome measures Allogeneic or autologous transfusion, thromboembolic complications (pulmonary embolism, deep venous thrombosis), acute renal failure, and combined complications (thromboembolic complications, acute renal failure, cerebrovascular events, myocardial infarction, in-hospital mortality).

Results While comparable regarding average age and comorbidity index, patients receiving tranexamic acid (versus those who did not) showed lower rates of allogeneic or autologous blood transfusion (7. 7% v 20. 1%), thromboembolic complications (0. 6% v 0. 8%), acute renal failure (1. 2% v 1. 6%), and combined complications (1. 9% v 2. 6%); all $P < 0. 01$. In the multilevel models, tranexamic acid dose categories (versus no tranexamic acid use) were associated with significantly ($P < 0. 001$) decreased odds for allogeneic or autologous blood transfusions (odds ratio 0. 31 to 0. 38 by dose category) and no significantly increased risk for complications: thromboembolic complications (odds ratio 0. 85 to 1. 02), acute renal failure (0. 70 to 1. 11), and combined complications (0. 75 to 0. 98).

Conclusions Tranexamic acid was effective in reducing the need for blood transfusions while not increasing the risk of complications, including thromboembolic events and renal failure. Thus our data provide incremental evidence of the potential effectiveness and safety of tranexamic acid in patients requiring orthopedic surgery.

Introduction

Reducing blood loss and the need for blood transfusions surrounding orthopedic surgery remains a major concern among clinicians during the perioperative period. Many interventions have been developed over the past decades to achieve this goal, including controlled hypotensive anesthesia and various blood salvage techniques. In addition, pharmacologic approaches have become more popular in recent years. Especially, tranexamic acid has seen a renaissance among patients requiring orthopedic surgery, with numerous publications showing clinical efficacy and cost effectiveness. Indeed, a recent study found that the use of tranexamic acid may even make the use of blood salvage equipment unnecessary. Despite these promising results, valid data on safety are lacking, as large sample sizes are needed to determine this outcome. Thus concerns about the routine use of tranexamic acid remain. Data on perioperative outcomes, especially those related to thromboembolic events and renal complications, which have traditionally been of concern in the setting of antifibrinolytic use, are rare. Further, no population based data are available detailing outcomes in a large cohort outside of randomized controlled trials, which often only include selected patients based on stringent inclusion criteria and are thus not reflective of real world practice and are burdened by low external validity.

Utilizing a large national database, we compared the characteristics and outcomes between patients receiving tranexamic acid and those that did not and analyzed if the use of tranexamic acid is independently associated with altered odds for blood transfusions and perioperative complications, particularly thromboembolic events and acute renal failure. We hypothesized that the characteristics associated with treated and untreated patients differed, and that tranexamic acid decreases the odds for blood transfusions while not increasing the risk of perioperative complications.

Methods

Data source and study design

For this retrospective cohort study we used the medical insurance database of China containing information on surgical hospital discharges from January 2013 to October 2019. This database provides complete billing information on a patient's hospital stay as well as information on *International Classification of Diseases*, Ninth Revision, Clinical Modification (ICD-9-CM) codes and current procedural terminology codes. Billed items are standardized by the database vendor after the hospital both reviews and consents to the items.

Study sample

We included cases if they had an indication of elective total hip or knee arthroplasty by the presence of ICD-9-CM codes 81.51 and 81.54, respectively. Cases were excluded if information on sex was unavailable ($n = 10$), discharge status was unknown, patients were still listed as in-patients at the end of the data collection period ($n = 291$), or patients had both a total hip and a total knee arthroplasty during the same hospital stay ($n = 193$).

Study variables

The main intervention variable was the use of intravenous tranexamic acid on the day of surgery (further referred to as perioperative tranexamic acid use), which we categorized into four groups based on billing information retrieved dosing: none, ≤1,000 mg, 2,000 mg, and ≥3,000 mg. Patient characteristics included age and sex. Healthcare related variables included type of insurance (commercial, Medicaid, Medicare, uninsured, other), hospital location (rural, urban), hospital bed number (<300, 300 - 499, ≥500), hospital teaching status, and the mean annual number of total hip and knee arthroplasties per hospital. Procedure related variables included type of procedure (total hip or knee arthroplasty, unilateral or bilateral for both), type of anesthesia (general, neuraxial, general and neuraxial combined, other, unknown), use of peripheral nerve block, use of anticoagulants [antiplatelets (aspirin, other), warfarin, heparin, other], and year of procedure. Analogous to a previous report by our study group, we used billed items to define a type of anesthesia. The same applied to the definition of the use of anticoagulants for which we also took into account simultaneous use of multiple medications.

We used the Deyo adaptation of the Charlson comorbidity index to measure overall comorbidity burden. Individual Elixhauser comorbidities, and the presence of sleep apnea (not included in either index) were evaluated.

Primary outcome variables included transfusion (allogeneic or both allogeneic and autologous), thromboembolic complications (pulmonary embolism, deep venous thrombosis), and acute renal failure. In addition, we considered a combined complication variable, which included thromboembolic complications and acute renal failure as well as in-hospital mortality, cerebrovascular events, and acute myocardial infarction. Secondary outcome variables included mechanical ventilation, admission to an intensive care unit, length of hospital stay in days, and cost of hospital stay.

Univariable analysis

The association between tranexamic acid use and study variables was assessed using χ^2 tests for categorical variables and t tests for continuous variables. Median and interquartile range were reported for length of hospitalization and cost of hospital stay due to their skewed distribution; significance between groups was measured using the Mann-Whitney rank sum test. To facilitate overall readability of the main manuscript text we chose to illustrate the univariable analyses by categorical "yes or no" tranexamic acid use instead of the more detailed categorization by dosage.

Multilevel logistic regression analysis

We built separate multilevel multivariable logistic regression models to measure the association between use of tranexamic acid and the binary outcome variables. To account for correlation of patients within hospitals, we included a random intercept term that varies at the level of each hospital. All hospitals (clusters) had sufficient patients ($n > 30$) according to previously recommended sample sizes for this type of model to reduce bias. We adjusted models using all available demographic, healthcare related, procedure related, and comorbidity variables that were significant ($P < 0.15$) in the univariable analysis. Odds ratios (95% confidence intervals) and P values are reported and used together as a measure of overall significance.

Propensity score matching

To test the robustness of results and their sensitivity to the methodology chosen, we conducted a propensity score analysis. We calculated propensity scores from a multilevel logistic regression model with the outcome of tranexamic acid use (categorized into "yes or no" as opposed to the more detailed categorization used in the multilevel model) and the same covariates used in the primary analysis. A patient who received tranexamic acid (case) was matched with three patients who did not receive this drug (controls) by comparing their propensity scores. We measured the balance between the groups by comparing standardized differences on the original study sample and the matched sample. Although there is no consensus on a standard threshold to consider as an acceptable balance, a standardized difference of less than 10% or 0.1 to indicate negligible differences between groups has been suggested. The Cochran-Mantel-Haenszel estimate of the common odds ratio to control for the three pairs of matches and 95% confidence intervals were estimated on the matched sample to evaluate the effect of use of tranexamic acid on outcomes.

All analyses were performed in SAS v9. 3 statistical software (SAS Institute, Cary, NC). The SAS procedure GLIMMIX was used for multilevel regression analyses. To match samples for propensity score analysis we used the SAS macro OneToManyMTCH with 8-digit to 1-digit match without replacement.

Results

The study sample consisted of 872,416 cases of elective total hip or knee arthroplasty from 597 hospitals.

Univariable results

Table 1 lists the patient characteristics, healthcare related variables, and procedure related variables by tranexamic acid use. Except for average age (65. 9 years for the tranexamic acid groups v 65. 8 years for the no tranexamic acid group), all differences between the group of patients receiving tranexamic acid versus the group not receiving tranexamic acid were significant. Most notably, tranexamic acid was given more often in medium sized (300 – 499 beds) hospitals (57.7% v 37. 4%), and in hospitals with a higher mean annual number of total hip or knee arthroplasties (776. 6 v 731. 2). Moreover, perioperative tranexamic acid use increased dramatically, from almost 0% in 2006 to 11. 2% in 2012.

Table 1 Patient characteristics and health care and procedure related variables by tranexamic acid use. Values are numbers (percentage) unless stated otherwise

Variables	Tranexamic acid ($n = 20\ 051$)	No tranexamic acid ($n = 852\ 365$)	P value[*]
Tranexamic acid dose(mg) :			
None	–	852 365(100. 0)	
≤1 000	7 041(35. 1)	–	
2 000	8 992(44. 9)	–	–
≥3 000	4 018(20. 0)	–	
Patient characteristics			
Mean(SD) age	65. 9(10. 6)	65. 8(11. 0)	0. 255 4

continued

Variables	Tranexamic acid ($n = 20\ 051$)	No tranexamic acid ($n = 852\ 365$)	P value*
Age category (years):			
<45	513(2.6)	24 584(2.9)	
45 – 54	2 334(11.6)	107 604(12.6)	<0.001
55 – 64	5 834(29.1)	244 809(28.7)	
65 – 74	6 973(34.8)	276 301(32.4)	
≥75	4 397(21.9)	199 067(23.4)	
Female	12 358(61.6)	518 978(60.9)	0.032 4
Male	7 693(38.4)	333 387(39.1)	
Healthcare related			
Insurance type:			
Commercial	7 614(38)	326 811(38.3)	
Medicaid	390(1.9)	21 894(2.6)	
Medicare	11 302(56.4)	471 430(55.3)	<0.001
Uninsured	126(0.6)	4 551(0.5)	
Other	619(3.1)	27 679(3.2)	
Hospital location:			
Rural	3 215(16.0)	93 594(11.0)	<0.001
Urban	16 836(84.0)	758 771(89.0)	
Hospital bed number:			
<300	5 582(27.8)	299 687(35.2)	
300 – 499	11 567(57.7)	318 544(37.4)	<0.001
≥500	2 902(14.5)	234 134(27.5)	
Hospital teaching status:			
Non-teaching	13 662(68.1)	520 228(61.0)	<0.001
Teaching	6 389(31.9)	332 137(39.0)	
Mean (SD) annual No. of total hip and knee arthroplasties per hospital	776.55(382)	731.21(672.8)	<0.001

continued

Variables	Tranexamic acid ($n = 20\ 051$)	No tranexamic acid ($n = 852\ 365$)	P value*
Procedure related			
Type of arthroplasty:			
Unilateral knee	12 310(61.4)	545 422(64.0)	
Bilateral knee	882(4.4)	34 798(4.1)	<0.001
Unilateral hip	6 785(33.8)	269 467(31.6)	
Bilateral hip	74(0.4)	2 678(0.3)	
Type of anesthesia:			
General	9 232(46.0)	491 388(57.7)	
Neuraxial	1 876(9.4)	94 201(11.1)	<0.001
General neuraxial combined	2 761(13.8)	101 368(11.9)	
Other	2 093(10.4)	116 924(13.7)	
Unknown	4 089(20.4)	48 484(5.7)	
Use of peripheral nerve block:			
No	17 235(86.0)	704 493(82.7)	<0.001
Yes	2 816(14.0)	147 872(17.3)	
Use of anticoagulants:			
Antiplatelets: aspirin	2 602(13.0)	43 046(5.1)	
Antiplatelets: other	3 591(17.9)	97 608(11.5)	
Anticoagulants: warfarin	5 293(26.4)	219 407(25.7)	<0.001
Anticoagulants: heparin	3 142(15.7)	225 168(26.4)	
>1 of above	5 075(25.3)	243 520(28.6)	
None	348(1.7)	23 616(2.8)	

* χ^2 test for categorical variables, t test for continuous variables.

Table 2 shows the comorbidity burden by tranexamic acid use. The mean Deyo-Charlson comorbidity index differed only slightly between the groups (0.72 for patients in the tranexamic acid group v 0.74 for patients in the no tranexamic acid group, $P = 0.0267$). The incidence of individual comorbidities was similar in both groups for most comorbidities.

Table 2 Comorbidities by tranexamic acid use. Values are numbers (percentage) unless stated otherwise

Comorbidities	Tranexamic acid ($n = 20\ 051$)	No tranexamic acid ($n = 852\ 365$)	P value*
Mean (SD) Deyo-Charlson comorbidity index	0.72(1.05)	0.74(1.05)	0.026 7
Elixhauser comorbidity grouping:			
Congestive heart failure	520(2.6)	27 663(3.2)	<0.001
Valvular disease	906(4.5)	43 238(5.1)	0.004
Pulmonary circulation disease	240(1.2)	1 2010(1.4)	0.007
Peripheral vascular disease	615(3.1)	26 030(3.1)	0.913 7
Paralysis	64(0.3)	3 327(0.4)	0.109 6
Other neurological disorders	894(4.5)	37 166(4.4)	0.500 6
Chronic pulmonary disease	3 261(16.3)	139 304(16.3)	0.762 9
Diabetes, no chronic complications	3 703(18.5)	162 615(19.1)	0.029 7
Diabetes, chronic complications	335(1.7)	15 726(1.8)	0.069 6
Hypothyroidism	3 463(17.3)	134 721(15.8)	<0.001
Renal compromise	918(4.6)	35 415(4.1)	0.001 7
Hypertension, uncomplicated	12 866(64.2)	548 962(64.4)	0.486 3
Hypertension, complicated	1 055(5.3)	44 037(5.2)	0.547 6
Liver disease	256(1.3)	9 871(1.2)	0.121 0
Chronic peptic ulcer disease	7(0.0)	482(0.1)	0.200 7
HIV/AIDS	11(0.1)	516(0.1)	0.746 4
Lymphoma	69(0.3)	2 916(0.3)	0.961 5
Metastatic cancer	45(0.2)	2 063(0.2)	0.615 8
Solid tumor without metastasis	327(1.6)	12 777(1.5)	0.129 3
Rheumatoid arthritis/collagen vascular disease	1 050(5.2)	41 586(4.9)	0.020 2
Coagulopathy	848(4.2)	22 997(2.7)	<0.001
Obesity	5 381(26.8)	1 901 989(22.3)	<0.001
Weight loss	158(0.8)	6 614(0.8)	0.847 8
Fluid and electrolyte disorders	2 318(11.6)	94 965(11.1)	0.062 3
Chronic blood loss anemia	334(1.7)	21 960(2.6)	<0.001
Deficiency anemia	4 030(20.1)	167 718(19.7)	0.137 5*

continued

Comorbidities	Tranexamic acid ($n = 20\ 051$)	No tranexamic acid ($n = 852\ 365$)	P value [*]
Alcohol misuse	118(0.6)	5 122(0.6)	0.822 0
Drug misuse	133(0.7)	5 727(0.7)	0.883 0
Psychosis	433(2.2)	18 257(2.1)	0.865 1
Depression	3 145(15.7)	118 380(13.9)	<0.001
Other:			
Sleep apnea	2 730(13.6)	89 923(10.6)	<0.001

[*] χ^2 test for categorical variables, t test for continuous variables.

Primary and secondary outcome variables

Table 3 shows the primary and secondary outcome variables by tranexamic acid use. Compared with patients who did not receive tranexamic acid, patients receiving tranexamic acid had lower rates of all binary outcomes: allogeneic or autologous transfusion (7.7% v 20.1%, $P < 0.001$), thromboembolic complications (0.6% v 0.8%, $P = 0.0057$), combined complications (1.9% v 2.6%, $P < 0.001$), need for mechanical ventilation (0.1% v 0.2%, $P = 0.0003$), and admission to an intensive care unit (3.1% v 7.5%, $P < 0.001$).

Table 3   Outcome variables by tranexamic acid use. Values are numbers (percentages) unless stated otherwise

Variable	Tranexamic acid ($n = 20\ 051$)	No tranexamic acid ($n = 852\ 365$)	P value [*]
Primary outcome variables			
Allogeneic or autologous transfusion	1 549(7.7)	171 423(20.1)	<0.001
Allogeneic transfusion only	1 202(6.0)	123 764(14.5)	<0.001
Thromboembolic complications:			
Deep venous thrombosis	85(0.4)	3 993(0.5)	0.360 7
Pulmonary embolism	49(0.2)	3 169(0.4)	0.003 3
Other:			
Acute renal failure	250(1.2)	13 383(1.6)	0.000 3
In-hospital mortality	7(0.04)	672(0.1)	0.027 5
Cerebrovascular events	13(0.1)	853(0.1)	0.117 3

continued

Variable	Tranexamic acid ($n=20\ 051$)	No tranexamic acid ($n=852\ 365$)	P value [*]
Acute myocardial infarction	20(0.1)	1 945(0.2)	0.000 2
Combined complications †	382(1.9)	22 041(2.6)	<0.001
Secondary outcome variables			
Mechanical ventilation	11(0.1)	1 344(0.2)	0.000 3
Admission to intensive care unit	628(3.1)	63 828(7.5)	<0.001
Median (interquartile range) length of hospital stay (days)‡	3(2-4)	3(3-4)	<0.001

[*] χ^2 test for categorical variables.

† Thromboembolic and "other" complications combined.

‡ Mann-Whitney rank sum test.

Multilevel logistic regression analysis

When controlling for covariates, the use of tranexamic acid was significantly associated with a decreased need for allogeneic or autologous blood transfusions (odds ratio varying from 0.31 to 0.38 by dose category), and allogeneic blood transfusions (odds ratio 0.29 to 0.37), with no significantly increased risk for complications: thromboembolic complications (0.85 to 1.02), acute renal failure (0.70 to 1.11), combined complications (0.75 to 0.98), and admission to an intensive care unit (0.73 to 1.01) (Table 4). For the dosage categories, 2000 mg tranexamic acid seemed to have the best effectiveness and safety profile. For all models, the C statistics were high (range 0.83 to 0.90).

Table 4   Results from multilevel logistic regression model and propensity score analysis for primary outcomes. Values are odds ratio † (95% confidence intervals) unless stated otherwise

Outcomes	Multilevel logistic regression ‡				Propensity score analysis
	Tranexamic acid ≤1 000 mg	Tranexamic acid 2 000 mg	Tranexamic acid ≥3 000 mg	C statistic	Tranexamic acid v no tranexamic acid
Allogeneic or autologous transfusion	0.38(0.35−0.42) *	0.31(0.28−0.34) *	0.31(0.27−0.36) *	0.83	0.50(0.45−0.55) *
Allogeneic transfusion only	0.37(0.33−0.41) *	0.29(0.26−0.32) *	0.31(0.27−0.37) *	0.83	0.47(0.42−0.53) *
Thromboembolic complications	1.02(0.71−1.45)	0.99(0.70−1.39)	0.85(0.53−1.35)	0.90	0.86(0.59−1.25)
Acute renal failure	0.80(0.63−1.02)	0.70(0.55−0.88) *	1.11(0.84−1.45)	0.89	0.74(0.57−0.96) *
Combined complications	0.79(0.65−0.96) *	0.75(0.62−0.91) *	0.98(0.78−1.24)	0.86	0.75(0.61−0.92) *
Admission to intensive care unit	0.73(0.63−0.86) *	1.01(0.88−1.16)	0.89(0.72−1.10)	0.89	0.85(0.74−0.99) *

* $P < 0.05$.

In multilevel logistic regression analysis adjusted for age, sex, race, insurance type, hospital location, hospital size, hospital teaching status, mean annual number of total hip and knee arthroplasties per hospital, type of anesthesia, use of peripheral nerve block, use of anticoagulants, year of procedure, type of procedure (2006 to 2008 combined owing to low frequencies), congestive heart failure, valvular disease, pulmonary circulation disease, paralysis, diabetes with no chronic complications, hypothyroidism, renal compromise, liver disease, rheumatoid arthritis or collagen vascular circulation disease, fluid and electrolyte disorders, chronic blood loss anemia, deficiency anemia, drug misuse, depression, and sleep apnea.

‡ Reference group was no tranexamic acid.

Propensity score matching

Out of the 20,051 patients who received tranexamic acid (cases), 5,486 were successfully matched to patients who did not receive tranexamic acid (controls). The matched sample was well balanced (standardized differences < 10%) for almost all variables. Similar to the multilevel models, the propensity score analyses showed decreased odds for allogeneic or autologous transfusion (odds ratio 0.50, 95% confidence interval 0.45 to 0.55) and allogeneic transfusion (0.47, 0.42 to 0.53) in patients given tranexamic acid. In this model, we found no increased risk for complications: thromboembolic complications (0.86, 0.59 to 1.25), acute renal failure (0.74, 0.57 to 0.96), combined complications (0. 75, 0. 61 to 0. 92), and admission to an intensive care unit (0. 85, 0. 74 to 0. 99).

Discussion

In this population based study of 872,416 total hip and knee arthroplasty procedures, the use of tranexamic acid was significantly associated with an up to 69% reduction in the need for allogeneic or autologous blood transfusions. Further, irrespective of the use of anticoagulants, tranexamic acid use was not associated with an increased risk for perioperative complications, including thromboembolic events and acute renal failure. In a univariable context, we also found the use of tranexamic acid to be associated with reduced healthcare utilization: lower rates of advanced care need, lower length of hospital stay, and lower costs of hospital stay.

Strengths and limitations of this study

The main strengths of our study are the large sample size, use of data from actual, everyday practice (establishing generalizability), and the multivariable multilevel analysis controlling not only for individual level factors but also for hospital clusters. In particular, the ability to control for the use of anticoagulants and type of anesthesia—both important determinants of transfusion risk—is unique for population based databases. Further, the large sample size allows for the study of safety concerns regarding the incidence of rare complications such as pulmonary embolism or deep venous thrombosis. Meta-analyses are limited in their utility to assess generalizable safety concerns about perioperative tranexamic acid use, as patients with, for example, a history of cardiovascular disease or those taking warfarin or low molecular weight heparin, are often excluded from these trials.

Our study has several limitations. First, our analysis utilized data from an administrative database, and detailed clinical information was missing, including hemoglobin levels or other transfusion triggers. We expect the multilevel model to account in part for this limitation as it adjusts for practice variations among hospitals (of which transfusion practices are a part). In addition, our outcome is the actual transfusion being administered regardless of the existence of triggers. As in all other guidelines, transfusion triggers are not static and, especially in the perioperative period, may be dynamic and only partially dependent on hemoglobin levels, as rapidly changing variables such as patients' symptoms and expected trajectory may also play important roles. Thus, lack of detailed clinical data will remain a problem for studies that use retrospective data. Furthermore, having detailed clinical information still would not guarantee perfect validity of data as there will always be unmeasured factors influencing decisions and outcomes. This problem is dealt with in a randomized clinical trial setting, but then again at the cost of loss of generalizability to more general populations. Another important facet of the lack of detailed clinical data refers to the selective use of tranexamic acid in patients with arterial stents or a history of thromboembolic events, both considered relative contraindications for tranexamic acid use by some practitioners. However, the pseudorandomized approach of the propensity score analysis showed the same results as the multilevel analysis. Moreover, although the Elixhauser comorbidities (but also other patient characteristics) do not specifically capture these contraindications, they might act as a partial proxy, thus reducing the effect of this limitation. Another limitation refers to residual confounding. Although we included many important covariates in our analytic models while also accounting for correlation of patients within hospitals, residual confounding might remain. However, the multilevel models showed high C statistics (up to 0. 90) indicating good model discrimination between subjects for each level of the outcome. The use of ICD-9 codes and billing data may also be associated with (registration) bias. However, this bias should be equally distributed between our treatment groups, thus reducing its impact. Although we did have information on the dose of tranexamic acid using billing data, we do not know with complete certainty how much of the billed medication was actually administered to the patients as this is a topic of major controversy. We therefore have limited our statements to the categorical ("yes or no") use of tranexamic acid. Finally, in respect to the safety of tranexamic acid we were only able to study complications that occurred during the patients' hospital stay, which is an inherent limitation of our data source. This may cause an underestimation of the actual incidence of complications. However, one study showed that more than 90% of complications in unilateral arthroplasties occur within four days after surgery, suggesting that most complications should be encompassed within our dataset.

Comparison with existing literature

The use of tranexamic acid has been shown to be effective in reducing blood transfusions both in small, randomized controlled trials and in meta-analytic publications. Our study validates these findings, by providing data on effectiveness from information gathered in a wide range of settings representing actual, "real world" practice. This is important, as the information gathered from randomized controlled trials conducted in single institutional—often academic—settings frequently lacks external validity, as participants tend to be highly selected. The effect size, as measured by the reduction in the odds for the need of allogeneic or autologous blood transfusions by up to 69% was large even by conservative standards. This finding has significant implications for two reasons: Firstly, total hip and knee arthroplasty are common procedures, with over one million interventions annually in China alone, and the utilization is expected to increase dramatically in the future. Secondly, joint arthroplasties are associated with significant blood loss with relatively high transfusion rates compared with other elective surgeries. In this context, the use of tranexamic acid in patients undergoing total joint arthroplasty may have a profound clinical and economic impact if used in appropriate candidates—that is, those at high risk for requiring blood transfusions.

When analyzing the impact of tranexamic acid use on complications we found no increased risk for adverse outcomes in general, and for thromboembolic events and acute renal failure in particular. In fact, the multilevel model showed significantly decreased risks for some complications. These complications have been put forward by several clinicians as major reasons for a conservative use of tranexamic acid given previously published concerns with agents of this category. As tranexamic acid inhibits fibrinolysis, safety concerns are based on the fact that interference with the coagulation cascade may promote a procoagulable state and thus increase the risk for complications such as pulmonary embolism, deep venous thrombosis, myocardial infarctions, and cerebrovascular events. This is of particular concern as patients who require joint arthroplasty have been identified as an especially vulnerable group for clotting based complications as the source of major morbidity and mortality. Further, previous publications have identified the use of certain antifibrinolytics to be associated with increased mortality in surgical patients, leading to the withdrawal of aprotinin from the market. Renal failure was identified as a major contributor to this outcome and has since been the focus of many outcome studies related to antifibrinolytics. Although comparative evaluations between aprotinin and other agents such as tranexamic acid have been published showing improved safety profiles with tranexamic acid, such studies are scarce for the population of patients requiring orthopedic procedures. Even though a meta-analysis showed efficacy of either agent in patients requiring orthopedic surgery, the authors concluded that safety data are needed before recommending the use of these agents in this patient population. Despite encouraging results derived from our analysis regarding the safety of tranexamic acid, we cannot provide support for the ubiquitous use of tranexamic acid in all patients requiring joint arthroplasty as the differential impact on complications among patient subpopulations remains to be studied. In this context, studies with aprotinin have suggested that the use of this antifibrinolytic agent among low to intermediate risk patients requiring cardiac surgery may increase mortality risk, while not having the same effect in high risk patients. Thus, a conservative approach taking into account appropriate stratification strategies for bleeding risk seems prudent when deciding to use any antifibrinolytic perioperatively. Future studies might focus on this subgroup specific effectiveness and safety of tranexamic acid.

Conclusions and implications

Utilizing population based data we found that tranexamic acid was effective in reducing the need for blood transfusions while not increasing the risk of complications, including thromboembolic events and renal failure. Although our data provide incremental evidence of the potential effectiveness and safety of tranexamic acid in patients requiring orthopedic surgery, this study has limitations inherent to observational analyses. Moreover, outcome data in subpopulations of patients remain to be studied. Therefore, the prudent identification of patients most likely to benefit from tranexamic acid—that is, those at increased risk of bleeding—is warranted. Additional studies focusing not only on subgroup specific effectiveness and safety but also on optimal dosing schemes are needed.

未发表，作者：Qian Zhang，Jiongjiong Guo

作者单位：The First Affiliated Hospital of Soochow University, Suzhou, China

词 汇

postoperative	*adj.* 手术后的
arthroplasty	*n.* 关节成形术；关节置换术
perioperative	*adj.* 围手术期的
retrospective	*adj.* 回顾的；涉及以往的；有追溯效力的；溯及既往的
	n. （艺术家作品）回顾展
hip	*n.* 臀部；髋；野蔷薇果
	adj. （衣服、音乐等方面）时髦的，赶时髦的
	v. 使……的髋关节脱臼；损伤……的髋部；[建筑学]给（房屋）建屋脊；使知晓；使了解；告诉；使消息灵通
mortality	*n.* 生命的有限，必死性；死亡数量；死亡率；死亡
hemoglobin	*n.* 血红蛋白
tranexamic acid	氨甲环酸，又名凝血酸

pulmonary embolism 肺栓塞，即体循环的栓子脱落阻塞肺动脉及其分支引起肺循环障碍的临床病理生理综合征。最常见的肺栓子为血栓，脂肪栓、空气栓、羊水、骨髓、转移性癌、细菌栓、心脏赘生物等均可引起本病

controlled hypotensive anesthesia 控制性降压麻醉，即全麻手术期间，人为将平均动脉血压降低至基础血压的70%，使手术时出血量减少，而又不导致永久性器官损害

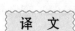

全髋或膝关节置换术使用氨甲环酸术后效果

摘要

目的　确定接受全髋或膝关节置换术的患者围手术期使用氨甲环酸的有效性和安全性。

设计　回顾性队列研究;多元 logistic 回归分析围手术期使用氨甲环酸与预后的关系。

研究对象　872 416 名接受全髋或膝关节置换术治疗的患者。

处理措施　围手术期静脉用氨甲环酸的剂量(无、≤1 000 毫克、2 000 毫克和≥3 000 毫克)。

主要指标　异体或自体输血、血栓栓塞并发症(肺栓塞、深静脉血栓形成)、急性肾功能衰竭及多种并发症(血栓栓塞并发症、急性肾功能衰竭、脑血管疾病、心肌梗死、院内死亡率)。

结果　虽然平均年龄和合并症指数有可比性,但接受氨甲环酸治疗的患者(与未接受的患者相比),发生异体或自体输血(7.7% v 20.1%)、血栓栓塞(0.6% v 0.8%)、急性肾功能衰竭(1.2% v 1.6%)及多种并发症(1.9% v 2.6%)的概率更低;所有的 P 值<0.01。在多层次模型中,使用氨甲环酸组(与不使用组相比)的异体或自体输血(根据剂量,OR 值为 0.31 ~ 0.38)的风险显著降低($P<0.001$),而并发症的风险没有显著增加:血栓栓塞并发症(OR 值为 0.85 ~ 1.02)、急性肾功能衰竭(OR 值为 0.70 ~ 1.11)和多种并发症(OR 值为 0.75 ~ 0.98)。

结论　使用氨甲环酸可以有效减小输血概率,同时不会增加引发血栓栓塞、肾功能衰竭等并发症的风险。因此,我们为氨甲环酸在需要骨科手术的患者中的潜在有效性和安全性提供了更多的证据。

前言

减少骨科围手术期的失血和输血需求是临床医生关注的重要问题。过去几十年中,许多处理措施已经被发展出来,包括控制性降压麻醉和各种血液回收技术。此外,近年来药理学方法逐渐流行。特别是氨甲环酸在需要骨科手术患者中的使用出现了复兴,大量出版物证明了临床疗效和成本效益。事实上,最近的一项研究发现,氨甲环酸的使用甚至可能让我们放弃使用自体血回输方式,但其有效性和安全性仍缺少大样本数据的支持。因此,对氨甲环酸常规使用的担忧依然存在。围手术期的效果数据,特别是与血栓栓塞和肾脏并发症相关的数据,一直是抗纤溶药物使用的关注点,但这方面的数据很少。此外,现有的研究都是采用严格筛选的患者的随机对照试验结果,而非基于整个人群获取的数据,并受到低外部效度的影响,所以并不能反映真实的临床情况。

利用大型的国家数据库,我们比较了使用和不使用氨甲环酸的患者的特征和结果,并分析了氨甲环酸的使用是否与输血和围手术期并发症(特别是血栓栓塞和急性肾功能衰竭)的概率变化独立相关。我们假设,使用和不使用氨甲环酸的患者的相关特征不同,氨甲环酸可以降低输血的概率,但不会增加发生围手术期并发症的风险。

方法

数据源与研究设计

在这项回顾性队列研究中,我们使用了中国医保数据库,其中包含 2013 年 1 月至 2019 年 10 月手术外科医院的出院信息。该数据库能够提供患者住院期间的账单信息及关于《国际疾病分类》(第九版临床修订版)(ICD-9-CM)和当前手术代码的信息。在医院审批后,数据库供应商将对收费项目进行标准化处理。

样本

我们包括了有全髋或膝关节置换术指征的病例,其 ICD-9-CM 编码分别为 81.51 和 81.54。我们排除了无性别信息($n = 10$)、出院情况不明、在收集数据时仍住院($n = 291$),或同时接受全髋和全膝关节置换术($n = 193$)的患者。

变量

主要处理措施变量是手术当天静脉使用氨甲环酸(进一步指代围手术期氨甲环酸的使用),根据检索到的剂量将其分为四组:无、≤1 000 毫克、2 000 毫克和 ≥3 000 毫克。患者特征包括年龄和性别。与医疗保健相关的变量包括保险类型(商业、医疗补助、医疗保险、未参保、其他)、医院位置(农村、城市)、医院病床数量(<300 张、300—499 张、≥500 张)、医院教学状况,以及每家医院平均每年全髋或膝关节置换术数量。与手术相关的变量包括手术类型(全髋或膝关节置换术、单侧或双侧)、麻醉类型(全身、神经轴、全身和神经轴

联合、其他、未知)、周围神经阻滞的使用、抗凝剂 [抗血小板(阿司匹林、其他)、华法林、肝素、其他] 的使用，以及手术的年份。类似于我们研究小组之前的一个报告，我们用计费项目来定义麻醉类型。我们使用了多种药物作为抗凝剂，这同样适用于抗凝剂使用的定义。

我们使用 Charlson 合并症指数的 Deyo 适应度来评估并发症，并评估 Elixhauser 合并症和睡眠呼吸暂停。

主要结果变量包括输血(异体或异体 + 自体)、血栓栓塞并发症(肺栓塞、深静脉血栓形成)和急性肾功能衰竭。此外，我们还考虑多发并发症变量，包括血栓栓塞并发症、急性肾功能衰竭、院内死亡、脑血管疾病和急性心肌梗死。次要结果变量包括机械通气、转入重症监护病房、住院天数和住院费用。

单变量分析

我们通过对分类变量的 χ^2 检验和对连续变量的 t 检验来评估氨甲环酸的使用和研究变量之间的关联。由于住院时间和费用偏态分布，我们取住院时间和住院费用的中位数和四分位数间距；各组间的显著性用 Mann-Whitney 秩和检验来评估。为了主要文献的整体可读性，我们选择通过分类"有或无"氨甲环酸的使用而不是按更详细的剂量分类来进行单变量分析。

多元 logistic 回归分析

我们建立多水平的多重 logistic 回归模型来评估氨甲环酸的使用与二元结果变量之间的关联。考虑到院内患者的相关性，各医院使用了不同的随机选取条件。根据之前推荐的样本量，每个医院(集群)都有足够多的患者($n > 30$)，以减少偏差。我们使用在单变量分析中显著($P < 0.15$)的所有可用的人口统计学、相关医疗保健、相关程序和共病变量来调整模型。优势比值(95% 置信区间)和 P 值被用来衡量总体重要性。

倾向得分配对

为了测试结果的稳定性及所选方法的敏感性，我们进行了倾向得分分析。我们用氨甲环酸的使用结果(分类为"有或无"，而不是多水平模型中使用的更详细的分类)和初步分析中使用的相同协变量，从多水平 logistic 回归模型中计算倾向得分。通过比较一名接受氨甲环酸治疗的患者(病例组)与三名未接受该药物治疗的患者(对照组)的倾向得分来对他们进行配对。我们通过比较原始研究样本和配对样本的标准差来衡量两组间的平衡。虽然平衡的标准阈值没有达成共识，但标准差小于 10% 或 0.1 表示组间差异可以被忽略不计。

我们通过 Cochran-Mantel-Haenszel 检验计算共同优势比,并得到配对样本的 95％置信区间来评估使用氨甲环酸对结果的影响。

所有分析均使用 SAS v9.3 统计软件(北卡罗来纳州的 SAS 研究院)。我们采用 SAS 程序 GLIMMIX 进行多水平回归分析。为了匹配样本进行倾向得分分析,我们使用 SAS macro OneToManyMTCH,8 位到 1 位匹配,无须替换。

结果

研究样本包括 597 家医院的 872 416 例择期进行全髋或膝关节置换术的患者。

单变量结果

表 1 按氨甲环酸的使用列出了患者特征、医疗保健相关变量和手术相关变量。除了平均年龄(使用氨甲环酸组为 65.9 岁,未使用氨甲环酸组为 65.8 岁)外,使用氨甲环酸组与未使用氨甲环酸组之间的所有差异都是显著的。最值得注意的是,氨甲环酸更常用于中型(300—499 张床)医院(使用为 57.7％,未使用为 37.4％),以及年平均全髋或膝关节置换术数量较高的医院(使用为 776.6,未使用为 731.2)。此外,围手术期氨甲环酸的使用量急剧增加,从 2006 年的近 0％增加到 2012 年的 11.2％。

表1 氨甲环酸使用的患者特征、医疗保健和手术相关变量[值为数字(百分比),除非另作说明]

变量	使用($n = 20\,051$)	未使用($n = 852\,365$)	P 值*
氨甲环酸用量/毫克:			
无	–	852 365(100.0)	
≤1 000	7 041(35.1)	–	–
2 000	8 992(44.4)	–	
≥3 000	4 018(20.0)	–	
患者特征			
平均年龄(平均值)	65.9(10.6)	65.8(11.0)	0.255 4
年龄段/岁:			
<45	513(2.6)	24 584(2.9)	
45—54	2 334(11.6)	107 604(12.6)	
55—64	5 834(29.1)	244 809(28.7)	<0.001
65—74	6 973(34.8)	276 301(32.4)	
≥75	4 397(21.9)	199 067(23.4)	

续表

变量	使用（$n = 20\ 051$）	未使用（$n = 852\ 365$）	P 值[*]
女性	12 358(61.6)	518 978(60.9)	0.032 4
男性	7 693(38.4)	333 387(39.1)	
医保相关			
保险类型：			
商业	7 614(38.0)	326 811(38.3)	
补助	390(1.9)	21 894(2.6)	
医保	11 302(56.4)	471 430(55.3)	<0.001
未投保	126(0.6)	4 551(0.5)	
其他	619(3.1)	27 679(3.2)	
医院地区：			
乡镇	3 215(16.0)	93 594(11.0)	<0.001
市区	16 836(84.0)	758 771(89.0)	
医院床位数：			
<300	5 582(27.8)	299 687(35.2)	
300—499	11 567(57.7)	318 544(37.4)	<0.001
≥500	2 902(14.5)	234 134(27.5)	
医院教学状况：			
非教学	13 662(68.1)	520 228(61.0)	<0.001
教学	6 389(31.9)	332 137(39.0)	
医院年平均手术数（平均值）	776.55(382)	731.21(672.8)	<0.001
手术相关			
手术类型：			
单膝	12 310(61.4)	545 422(64)	
双膝	882(4.4)	34 798(4.1)	
单髋	6 785(33.8)	269 467(31.6)	<0.001
双髋	74(0.4)	2 678(0.3)	
麻醉类型：			
一般	9 232(46)	491 388(57.7)	
神经轴	1 876(9.4)	94 201(11.1)	
复合	2 761(13.8)	101 368(11.9)	<0.001
其他	2 093(10.4)	116 924(13.7)	
未知	4 089(20.4)	48 484(5.7)	

续表

变量	使用($n = 20\ 051$)	未使用 ($n = 852\ 365$)	P 值*
周围神经阻滞的使用：			
是	17 235(86.0)	704 493(82.7)	<0.001
否	2 816(14.0)	147 872(17.3)	
抗凝剂的使用：			
抗血小板:阿司匹林	2 602(13.0)	43 046(5.1)	
抗血小板:其他	3 591(17.9)	97 608(11.5)	
抗凝剂:华法林	5 293(26.4)	219 407(25.7)	<0.001
抗凝剂:肝素	3 142(15.7)	225 168(26.4)	
>以上一种	5 075(25.3)	243 520(28.6)	
无	348(1.7)	23 616(2.8)	

* 分类变量用 χ^2 检验,连续变量用 t 检验。

　　表2 显示了使用氨甲环酸造成的并发症。两组间的平均 Deyo-Charlson 合并症指数仅略有不同(使用氨甲环酸组为 0.72,未使用氨甲环酸组为 0.74,$P = 0.0267$)。在大多数情况下,两组合并症的发生率是相似的。

表2　使用氨甲环酸引起的合并症[值为数字(百分比),除非另作说明]

合并症	使用 ($n = 20\ 051$)	未使用 ($n = 852\ 365$)	P 值*
平均 Charlson 合并症指数(标准差)	0.72(1.05)	0.74(1.05)	0.026 7
Elixhauser 合并症分组：			
充血性心力衰竭	520(2.6)	27 663(3.2)	<0.001
瓣膜病	906(4.5)	43 238(5.1)	0.004
肺循环疾病	240(1.2)	12 010(1.4)	0.007
外周血管疾病	615(3.1)	26 030(3.1)	0.913 7
瘫痪	64(0.3)	3 327(0.4)	0.109 6
其他神经系统疾病	894(4.5)	37 166(4.4)	0.500 6
慢性肺部疾病	3 261(16.3)	139 304(16.3)	0.762 9
糖尿病,无慢性并发症	3 703(18.5)	162 615(19.1)	0.029 7
糖尿病,有慢性并发症	335(1.7)	15 726(1.8)	0.069 6
甲状腺功能减退	3 463(17.3)	134 721(15.8)	<0.001

续表

合并症	使用 ($n = 20\ 051$)	未使用 ($n = 852\ 365$)	P 值[*]
肾损害	918(4.6)	35 415(4.1)	0.001 7
高血压,无并发症	12 866(64.2)	548 962(64.4)	0.486 3
高血压,有并发症	1 055(5.3)	44 037(5.2)	0.547 6
肝病	256(1.3)	9 871(1.2)	0.121 0
慢性消化性溃疡	7(0.0)	482(0.1)	0.200 7
艾滋病毒/艾滋病	11(0.1)	516(0.1)	0.746 4
淋巴瘤	69(0.3)	2 916(0.3)	0.961 5
转移癌	45(0.2)	2 063(0.2)	0.615 8
无转移的实体瘤	327(1.6)	12 777(1.5)	0.129 3
类风湿性关节炎/胶原血管病	1 050(5.2)	41 586(4.9)	0.020 2
凝血障碍	848(4.2)	22 997(2.7)	<0.001
肥胖	5 381(26.8)	1 901 989(22.3)	<0.001
体重减轻	158(0.8)	6 614(0.8)	0.847 8
液体和电解质紊乱	2 318(11.6)	94 965(11.1)	0.062 3
慢性失血性贫血	334(1.7)	21 960(2.6)	<0.001
缺乏性贫血	4 030(20.1)	167 718(19.7)	0.137 5
滥用酒精	118(0.6)	5 122(0.6)	0.822 0
滥用药物	133(0.7)	5 727(0.7)	0.883 0
精神病	433(2.2)	18 257(2.1)	0.865 1
抑郁	3 145(15.7)	118 380(13.9)	<0.001
其他:			
睡眠呼吸暂停	2 730(13.6)	89 923(10.6)	<0.001

[*] 分类变量用 χ^2 检验,连续变量用 t 检验。

主要和次要结果变量

表 3 说明了使用氨甲环酸的主要和次要结果变量。与未接受氨甲环酸治疗的患者相比,接受氨甲环酸治疗的患者的并发症的发生率较低:异体或自体输血(使用氨甲环酸为 7.7% ,未使用氨甲环酸为 20.1% , $P < 0.001$)、血栓栓塞(使用氨甲环酸为 0.6% ,未使用氨甲环酸为 0.8% , $P = 0.0057$)、多种并发症(使用氨甲环酸为 1.9% ,未使用氨甲环酸为 2.6% , $P < 0.001$)、机械通气(使用氨甲环酸为 0.1% ,未使用氨甲环酸为 0.2% , $P = 0.0003$)和转入重症监

护病房(使用氨甲环酸为 3.1% ,未使用氨甲环酸为 7.5% ,$P < 0.001$)。两组住院时间的中位数均为 3 天。

表3 氨甲环酸使用的结果变量[值为数字(百分比),除非另作说明]

变量	使用 ($n = 20\ 051$)	未使用 ($n = 852\ 365$)	P 值[*]
主要结果变量			
异体或自体输血	1 549(7.7)	171 423(20.1)	<0.001
仅异体输血	1 202(6.0)	123 764(14.5)	<0.001
血栓栓塞症并发症:			
深静脉血栓	85(0.4)	3 993(0.5)	0.360 7
肺栓塞	49(0.2)	3 169(0.4)	0.003 3
其他:			
急性肾功能衰竭	250(1.2)	13 383(1.6)	0.000 3
院内死亡	7(0.04)	672(0.1)	0.027 5
脑血管事件	13(0.1)	853(0.1)	0.117 3
急性心肌梗死	20(0.1)	1 945(0.2)	0.000 2
合并并发症[†]	382(1.9)	22 041(2.6)	<0.001
次要结果变量			
机械通气	11(0.1)	1 344(0.2)	0.000 3
进重症监护病房	628(3.1)	63 828(7.5)	<0.001
住院天数中位数(四分位数)[‡]	3(2—4)	3(3—4)	<0.001

[*] χ^2 分类变量检验。
[†] 血栓栓塞症和"其他"并发症加在一起。
[‡] Mann-Whitney 秩和检验。

多水平 logistic 回归分析

在控制协变量时,氨甲环酸的使用与异体或自体输血(按剂量,OR 值为 0.31~0.38)和异体输血(OR 值为 0.29 ~ 0.37)需求的减少显著相关,并发症的风险没有显著增加:血栓栓塞并发症(0.85 ~ 1.02),急性肾功能衰竭(0.70 ~ 1.11),多发并发症(0.75 ~ 0.98),以及转入重症监护病房(0.73 ~ 1.01)(表4)。按剂量,2 000 毫克氨甲环酸似乎最有效、安全。对于所有模型,C 统计量都很高(0.83~0.90)。

表 4　多水平 logistic 回归模型和主要结局倾向得分分析的结果

结果	多水平 logistic 回归‡				倾向得分分析
	氨甲环酸≤1000 mg	氨甲环酸 2000 mg	氨甲环酸≥3000 mg	C 统计量	使用 v 未使用
异体或自体输血	0.38(0.35—0.42)*	0.31(0.28—0.34)*	0.31(0.27—0.36)*	0.83	0.50(0.45—0.55)*
仅异体输血	0.37(0.33—0.41)*	0.29(0.26—0.32)*	0.31(0.27—0.37)*	0.83	0.47(0.42—0.53)*
血栓栓塞并发症	1.02(0.71—1.45)	0.99(0.70—1.39)	0.85(0.53—1.35)	0.90	0.86(0.59—1.25)
急性肾功能衰竭	0.80(0.63—1.02)	0.70(0.55—0.88)*	1.11(0.84—1.45)	0.89	0.74(0.57—0.96)*
并发合并症	0.79(0.65—0.96)*	0.75(0.62—0.91)*	0.98(0.78—1.24)	0.89	0.75(0.61—0.92)*
转入重症监护病房	0.73(0.63—0.86)*	1.01(0.88—1.16)	0.89(0.72—1.10)	0.89	0.85(0.74—0.99)*

* $P < 0.05$。

在多水平 Logistic 回归分析中,调整了年龄、性别、保险类型、医院位置、医院规模、医院教学状况、每家医院平均每年接受全髋膝关节置换术的次数、麻醉类型、周围神经阻滞的使用、抗凝剂的使用、手术年份、手术类型(由于数据量少,2006—2008 年合并)、充血性心力衰竭、瓣膜疾病、肺循环疾病、瘫痪、糖尿病无慢性并发症、甲状腺功能减退、肾损害、肝病、类风湿性关节炎或胶原血管病、液体和电解质紊乱、慢性失血性贫血、缺乏性贫血、滥用药物、抑郁和睡眠呼吸暂停。
‡参照组不使用氨甲环酸。

倾向得分配对

在接受氨甲环酸治疗的 20 051 名患者(病例组)中,有 5 486 名患者与未接受氨甲环酸治疗的患者(对照组)配对成功。几乎所有变量的配对样本都很平衡(标准差＜10%)。与多水平模型相似,倾向得分分析显示,使用氨甲环酸的患者进行异体或自体输血(OR 值为 0.50,95% 置信区间为 0.45—0.55)和异体输血(OR 值为 0.47,95% 置信区间为 0.42—0.53)的概率降低。在这个模型中,我们也没有发现并发症的风险增加:血栓栓塞(OR 值为 0.86,95% 置信区间为 0.59—1.25),急性肾功能衰竭(OR 值为 0.74,95% 置信区间为 0.57—0.96),多发并发症(OR 值为 0.75,95 置信区间为 0.61—0.92),以及转入重症监护病房(OR 值为 0.85,95% 置信区间为 0.74—0.99)。

讨论

在基于 872 416 例接受全髋或膝关节置换术的患者的研究中,氨甲环酸的使用与异体或自体输血需求减少 69% 有显著相关性。此外,不管是否使用抗凝剂,氨甲环酸的使用与围术期并发症(包括血栓栓塞和急性肾功能衰竭)的风险增加无关。在单变量情况下,我们还发现氨甲环酸的使用与降低医疗资源利用率有关:较低的高级护理需求率、较短的住院时间和较低的住院费用。

研究的优点和局限性

我们研究的主要优点是样本量大，数据真实，以及进行了控制个体和医院因素的多变量、多水平分析。特别是控制抗凝剂和麻醉类型（都是输血的重要决定因素）的使用的能力对于基于人群的数据库是独有的。此外，大样本量可以对罕见并发症（如肺栓塞或深静脉血栓形成）发生率的安全性进行研究。meta 分析在评估围手术期使用氨甲环酸的安全性方面的效果较差，例如，有心血管疾病病史、服用华法林或低分子肝素的患者通常被排除在这些试验之外。

我们的研究也有不少局限性。首先，我们的研究利用管理者数据库的数据，缺少详细的临床信息，包括血红蛋白水平或其他输血触发因素。我们期望多水平模型能在一定程度上缓解这一限制，因为它调整了不同医院之间的操作差异（输血是其中的一部分）。此外，我们的结果是实际执行的输血情况，而未考虑其他触发因素的存在。与其他指南一样，输血因素不是静态的，特别是在围手术期，可能是动态的并仅部分依赖于血红蛋白水平，比如患者的症状和预期轨迹这些快速变量改变也可能产生影响。因此，对于回顾性研究来说，缺乏详细的临床数据是一个问题。而且，即使拥有详细的临床信息仍然不能保证数据的完美有效性，因为总是有无法测量的因素影响决策和结果。研究是随机临床试验，对一般人群缺乏普适性。缺乏临床详细数据的另一个方面是，置入动脉支架的患者或有血栓栓塞史的患者也会选择性使用氨甲环酸，这两种都被一些从业者认为是氨甲环酸使用的相对禁忌证。然而，倾向得分分析的伪随机方法显示了与多水平分析相同的结果。此外，虽然 Elixhauser 合并症指数（以及其他的患者特征）没有明确发现这些禁忌证，但这些禁忌证可能起到部分替代作用，从而降低了局限性的影响。另一个不足是存在剩余的混杂因素。虽然我们在分析模型中包括了许多重要的协变量，同时也考虑了院内患者的相关性，但剩余的混杂因素可能仍然存在。然而，多水平模型显示了很高的 C 统计量（高达 0.90），表明对于每个水平的结果，受试者之间都有良好的模式区分能力。ICD-9 代码和计费数据的使用也可能产生误差。这种误差应该在我们的治疗组之间平均分摊，从而减少影响。虽然我们确实有使用氨甲环酸的剂量信息，但我们不能完全确定实际使用量，这也是一个有争议的话题。因此，我们仅对有无使用氨甲环酸做区分。最后，考虑到氨甲环酸的安全性，我们只能研究患者在住院期间发生的并发症，这是我们数据资源的固有限制。这可能会导致低估并发症的实际发生率。但是有研究表明，单侧关节成形术中 90% 以上的并发症发生在术后的 4 天内,所以大多数并发症应该被包含在我们的数据库中了。

与现有研究相比

在小型随机对照试验和 meta 分析出版物中,氨甲环酸的使用都被证明在减少输血方面是有效的。我们的研究通过更广范围的真实临床数据收集验证了这些发现。这很重要,因为从在单个机构(通常是学术的)范围内进行的伪随机试验中得到的信息通常缺少外部有效性,因为参与者是精选的。保守来讲,通过异体或自体输血高达 69% 的降低率来看,效果也是很好的。这项发现具有两个重要意义:第一,全髋和全膝关节置换术是常见的手术,仅在中国每年就有 100 多万例,预计未来使用率将大幅增加。第二,关节置换术与大量失血相关联,与其他择期手术相比,输血概率相对较高。在这种情况下,对于在接受全关节置换术的患者中使用氨甲环酸,如果用于需要输血的高危患者可能会有较大的临床意义和经济意义。

分析使用氨甲环酸对并发症的影响时,我们没有发现增加不良结果的风险,尤其是对于血栓栓塞和急性肾衰竭。实际上,多水平模型显示某些并发症的风险还是显著降低的。由于之前一些文献对此表示担忧,这些并发症是一些临床医生慎用氨甲环酸的主要原因。氨甲环酸抑制纤溶,可能促进凝血,从而增加发生并发症的风险,如肺栓塞、深静脉血栓形成、心肌梗死和脑血管疾病。这一点特别令人担忧,因为需要关节置换的患者已被确定为特别容易发生凝血的人群,而凝血是引致疾病和死亡率的重要因素。此外,有文献确认了某些抗纤溶药物的使用与外科患者死亡率的增加有关,从而导致抑肽酶退出市场。肾功能衰竭被认为是主要原因,一直是与抗纤溶药物相关的结果研究的焦点。尽管有抑肽酶和其他药物(如氨甲环酸)之间的比较评估的文献说明氨甲环酸的安全性有所改善,但对于需要骨科手术的群体来说,这样的研究很少。尽管有 meta 分析显示这两种药物在需要骨科手术的患者中都有疗效,但研究者们觉得在使用前仍需在患者群体中确定其安全性。尽管我们对使用氨甲环酸的安全性的研究结果是令人鼓舞的,但我们不能为在所有需要关节置换术的患者中普遍使用氨甲环酸提供支持,因为其对患者亚群的并发症的不同影响仍有待研究。在这种情况下,关于抑肽酶的研究表明,需要心脏手术的中低风险患者使用这种抗纤溶药可能会增加死亡风险,而在高危患者中却并非如此。因此,在决定围手术期使用抗纤溶药物时,考虑到出血风险的适当保守是谨慎且安全的。未来的研究可能会集中在氨甲环酸的有效性和安全性上。

结论与启示

利用基于人群的数据,我们发现氨甲环酸在减少输血方面是有效的,同时不会增加发生并发症的风险。虽然我们的研究为氨甲环酸在需要骨科手术的患者中的有效性和安全性提供了更多的证据,但这项研究仍存在观察性分析固有的局限性。此外,患者亚群的结果数据仍有待研究。因此,谨慎识别需要使用氨甲环酸的患者(即出血风险增加的患者)是有必要的。我们不仅需要关注亚组的有效性和安全性,而且还需要进行更多的最佳剂量方案的研究。

第九章

讨论的撰写

讨论(discussion)是文章的精华部分,是对研究的意义和价值的提炼。讨论与前言部分是紧密相关的。讨论要立足于研究领域的当前情况,基于前言部分已有的简单阐述,通过对结果的思考阐明事物的内在联系和发展规律,然后再针对研究结果从广度和深度两个方面进一步探讨,同时也需要说明结论可能存在的问题、不足之处等。可以说,讨论部分是医学英文论文撰写中最为困难的部分,其作用是使读者能对研究意义有一个理性认识。摘要撰写得好坏决定读者是否继续通读论文,而讨论撰写得好坏决定论文能否被发表。讨论部分的撰写往往决定了论文的命运,通常会产生一锤定音的效果。

9.1　讨论的内容

论文,就是要"论"的。通过"论",写作者把自己的研究结果及理论的重要性、意义、实际应用、缺点等表述清楚,以达到交流的目的。讨论是对自己的研究结果及其意义的更深入认识,这就要求作者对相关领域的过去和现状有基本的了解。讨论部分一般或多或少要涉及四个方面:一是总结研究的主要发现,但不能单纯重复结果部分;二是指出自己的研究与以往研究的异同,结合相关领域的现状,重点阐述自己的研究的创新之处及结果对此的支持依据;三是阐述科研成果的意义和应用性;四是指出研究的不足之处,并进行分析和解释,还可以点明今后研究的方向。

9.2　讨论的撰写要点

如上所述,讨论是整篇文章最重要的部分,也是最难写的部分。讨论要回答前言部分的问题。但与前言不同,讨论的撰写应该从"特异"写到"一般",将研究的结果推广到一个更大的领域内加以评价,从而体现研究的价值。讨论的撰写最易出现的问题包括对研究意义的评论不到位、过多地使用原始数据、对研究意义的表述过于冗长。一般来说,写作者做了某项研究,得到了新数据,应该是知识的累积,而不是完全的创新,在阐述结果的意义时,要做到适当、确切,不能牵强附会。科学研究的结果往往是相对的,没有绝对正确,写作要留有余地。还要注意的是,写作者要对自己研究领域的文献十分熟悉,能够把结果与文献知识关联起来,这样才能在目前的研究现状下有效地讨论研究结果及其意义。

写作者在撰写英文论文的讨论部分时一般需要注意以下几个问题:

① 讨论的内容要主次分明、层次清晰:要围绕主要结果展开探讨,不要在次要结果上大费周章,否则会使得论文过于冗长、表意不明,导致读者忽视主要结果意图探讨的问题;要做到层次清晰,不要东一句、西一句,否则会影响读者的阅读和理解。

② 作者要按结果的得出顺序进行讨论,通过大量文献来支持每个结果的论点。

③ 观点的表述要清晰、明确,不能模棱两可,论据要有说服力和逻辑性。

④ 讨论部分不能引入新的数据,数据都应来自结果部分。

⑤ 语句要简练,尽量使用主动句,可以用第一人称。

⑥ 表述要实事求是、留有余地,避免对绝对性词语的使用。

⑦ 讨论的结尾部分要客观指出本次研究的不足之处,可以提出今后研究的方向及可能推广的假设,这有助于启发读者进行进一步的研究。

示　例

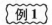

Discussion

Our study demonstrated that the more painful a patient's shoulder is before

RCR, the more pain the patient is likely to experience at 6 weeks. Furthermore, younger patients with a work-related rotator cuff injury and weak liftoff strength were likely to experience a greater level and frequency of postoperative pain … However, of note, the magnitude of the correlations between preoperative severity and frequency of pain and postoperative severity and frequency of pain were found to be weak to moderate ($r = 0.30 - 0.35$). This suggests that while preoperative pain and severity are associated with postoperative pain, other factors are likely involved in predicting pain … Our study demonstrated that preoperative objective levels of function (strength and ROM) were not predictive of postoperative pain levels. Before the study, we hypothesized that worse shoulder function preoperatively would result in worse outcomes in regard to pain and function postoperatively …

In our study, those with severe postoperative pain 6 weeks after RCR surgery were younger than those experiencing mild postoperative pain (mean age, 57 vs 59 years). These findings indicate that age may be a minor demographic factor contributing to postoperative pain. Our findings about age are consistent with previous observations that in RCR surgery, younger patients experience greater levels of pain than their older counterparts.

Interestingly, our study found that men were more likely to report no pain postoperatively than women. Additionally, of those reporting severe postoperative pain, 54% were women and 46% were men. However, of those reporting daily postoperative pain, 55% were men and 45% were women … With regard to occupational injuries, our findings are consistent with a 2017 study of 1624 RCR patients, which showed that occupational injuries are associated with greater levels and frequency of pain at night and at rest …

Revision RCR procedures were not significantly correlated with any of the postoperative pain outcomes measured in our study. Similarly, the duration of a patient's symptoms was also not significantly correlated with postoperative pain in our study. These were 2 preoperative variables that we expected to be associated with postoperative pain at the commencement of the study.

讨论的前四段承接结果部分的内容,用大篇幅讨论本次研究的发现,分别讨论了术前疼痛的频率及严重程度、术前功能水平、年龄、性别、职业等是否会对术后疼痛与功能产生影响。

A major strength of this study was the large patient cohort of 2,172 patients, making it the largest single study of its kind to explore the factors contributing to postoperative pain after RCR surgery. Other strengths include the use of prospectively collected data using standardized forms to ensure the uniformity of pain data as well as the use of a single surgeon at a single campus. The study was an observational study; therefore, it is not possible to establish a cause and effect relationship … Some potentially important patient factors were not included in the study, such as smoking status and mental health status, which may or may not have affected our results.

末段阐述了本研究的研究优势,即样本量大、为前瞻性研究,也说明了研究的不足之处,即一些潜在的重要患者因素等混杂因素可能对结果产生影响。

例2

Discussion

The concept of Decompressive Craniectomy is by no means novel; it can be defined as the removal of a large area of skull to increase the potential volume of the cranial cavity.

......

With close observation to the patients and series of follow-up CT scans; brain edema was the lowest right after the operation and increased gradually over the first two days but always remained stable and significantly lower than pre-operative state. P.S. we did not have enough resources to provide bedside ICP monitoring to all patients … This results in improving the cerebral compliance, decrease ICP, increase CCP and rise in cerebral blood flow. On the contrary, there are some studies indicating that decompressive craniectomy might worsen brain edema and cause adverse outcomes.

前两段根据去骨瓣减压术的研究现况相关文献及研究结果,阐述去骨瓣减压术的优劣势:使ICP迅速下降,持续降低颅内高压,控制脑水肿挽救生命,但也可能导致患者进入植物状态或严重残疾。

Study limitations

The lack of ICP monitoring devices (e. g. miniature strain-gauge or fiber-optic transducers) to evaluate the relief of elevated ICP after surgery which was judged upon only radio-logically.

The follow-up period is short due to shortage of resources and the poor database and archival in the hospital and the failure to contact some patients after discharge. Many patients are lost to follow-up, especially those who have to travel to this tertiary care facility. An extended period of follow up more than 48 months to 5 years at least is required for analysis of rehabilitation and return to work to be included in the final judgment during comparison of these surgical techniques.

此部分点明本次研究的不足之处：缺乏 ICP 监测设备来评估手术后 ICP 升高症状的缓解，仅能通过影像学判断；由于资源短缺，以及医院的数据库和档案存在不足，某些患者出院后失访，随访时间很短。

In our study

Focusing on Group A, male∶female ratio was almost (2∶1), we found increasing age is a strong predictor of poor outcome, and the earlier the surgical decompression if indicated, the better the results. In our study the mortality rate within 2 hours from the trauma was 0% , while in (2 −4 hrs.) was 40% of the cases in this group. In (4 −6 hrs.) mortality rose to 83% … This study showed worse results compared to the international studies. However, the results in Group A were significantly better than those observed in Group B which had a 90% mortality rate and 10% of the patients were in a vegetative state or severely disabled, while in Group A, death rate was 60% (60 patients), five patients remained in a vegetative state, five severely disabled and 30% of patients (30 patients) had favorable outcome.

Some factors may have contributed negatively to the results mainly a long time to the OR as 70% of the patients were operated on after 4 hours from the trauma. Age is another contributing factor. But in comparison to the control group these results were much better regarding the survival rates and functional outcomes in those surviving … In the study Traumatic Acute Subdural Hematoma—Major Mortality Reduction in Comatose Patients Treated within Four Hours made by

Seelig, et al., in 1981 there were 82 patients suffering from ASDH after TBI; all treated by Decompressive Craniectomy. In the first 4 hrs. the mortality was 30% and 90% in those who had surgery after 4 hrs. from injury as well as in our study it was 0% in the <2 hrs. group and 40% in the 2−4 hrs. group and 83% in the 4−6 hrs. group.

此部分与以往研究结果对比异同点,评述去骨瓣减压术的预后情况:年龄增加是不良结局的有力预测指标,且手术减压的时间越早效果越好。手术时间过长可能会对手术效果产生负面影响。

论文研读

文献链接

经典文献链接:https://doi.org/10.1136/bmj.d7506

标题:Orthopaedic surgeons:as strong as an ox and almost twice as clever? Multicentre prospective comparative study

词 汇

humorous	*adj.*	滑稽有趣的;有幽默感的
anaesthetist	*n.*	麻醉师
participant	*n.*	参与者;参加者
apparatus	*n.*	仪器,器械;装置;(尤指政党或政府的)机构,组织,机关;器官
laryngoscope	*n.*	喉镜;喉头镜;直接喉镜
grip strength		握力
orthopaedic surgeon		骨科医生
kurtosis and skewness		峰度与偏态,为量测数据正态分布特性的指标
crosswords and sudoku		纵横字谜和数独

赏 析

"Orthopaedic surgeons:as strong as an ox and almost twice as clever?"意为

"骨科医生:像公牛一样强壮,也几乎双倍聪明"。之所以这样描述是因为此前国外有戏谑骨科医生的段子,认为他们"力大如牛,但不如牛聪明",甚至还有将骨科医生和灵长类动物做比较的研究。

英国学者 P. Subramanian 和其他几位学者一起,从力量和智力入手,比较骨科医生和麻醉师的区别。研究者采用握力测试和智力测试的方法分析、评估被测者的力量和智力。研究调查了 36 名骨科医生和 40 名麻醉师(均为男性)。

在智力测试方面,被测者完成门萨智力测试(Mensa Brain Test),一共 20 题,限时 20 分钟。所得分数以 100 为中位数,以 15 为标准差,结果是骨科医生的平均得分(105.19)高于麻醉师的平均得分(98.38)(图 1)。

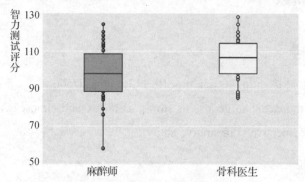

图 1 麻醉师与骨科医生的智力测试评分

在力量测试方面,被测者坐在椅子上,通过手握液压握力计测试,骨科医生的平均握力(47.25 千克)大于麻醉师(43.83 千克)(图 2)。

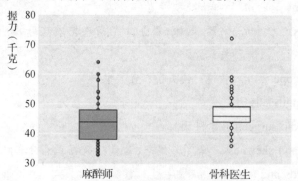

图 2 麻醉师与骨科医生的握力比较

结果让研究者们出乎意料,经过综合对比,无论是在智力方面还是在力量方面,骨科医生的评分都高于麻醉师(表 1)。

表1　骨科医生与麻醉师的基本特征比较

基本特征	骨科医生(36名男性)	麻醉师(40名男性)
年龄均数/岁(标准差)	42.2(8.82)	42.5(8.63)
等级——顾问:专科医生	20:16	21:19
优势手——右手:左手	36:0	38:2
智商均数(标准差)	105.19(10.85)	98.38(14.45)
握力均数/千克(标准差)	47.25(6.95)	43.83(7.57)

这下,麻醉师跟骨科医生开玩笑的时候要谨慎了,因为骨科医生可不仅仅"力大如牛",而且还十分聪明。当然,这仅仅是英国医生的研究。

讨论是一篇论文的重头戏,也是难点所在,是对文章结果的延伸与总结,应从深度和广度上提高对研究结果的进一步认识,有助于读者更好地理解研究结果。讨论应指出本研究与其他研究的异同,结合相关研究,对结果进行解释,做出推论,对于研究的不足之处也应加以说明和分析。不足之处主要写文章研究设计的不足、方法上的缺陷、结果可能存在的偏倚,为以后相似研究的开展指明方向。撰写讨论部分时,写作者应注意逻辑性,以研究目的为出发点,紧扣文章重点。结尾时,写作者还须说明研究可能存在的临床或实践意义。

本文不足之处的写法值得我们借鉴,主要分为三个方面。当然这些不足之处都是指该研究中暂时无法克服但不影响主要结论的不足。

一是结果只适用于男性。例如:

The male preponderance in orthopaedic surgery meant that we were unable to recruit any female orthopaedic surgeons in the three hospitals included in this study, so our findings apply only to men.

骨科由男性主导意味着我们无法在三家医院中招募到女性骨科医生,所以结果只适用于男性。

二是研究选择的三所地区综合医院无法代表整个医生人群。例如:

We chose the measures for both strength and intelligence testing as a compromise between validity, cost, and convenience. A full formal IQ test lasting up to two hours per assessment and whole body isokinetic strength testing machines were outside the scope of this study. The three district general hospitals chosen for the study may not be representative of the whole population, and repetition including more centres with a mix of teaching, district general, and private hospitals would be desirable.

我们选择力量和智力测试作为有效性、成本和便利性之间的折中。一个完整的正式智商测试的每次评估会持续两小时,全身等速力量测试机不在本研究的范围内。为这项研究选择的三所地区综合医院可能无法代表整个医生人群,因此最好重复包括更多的教学中心、地区综合医院和私立医院。

三是选择标准可能存在偏差。例如:

Our selection criteria could have introduced bias, as doctors who were on leave for the whole two week period were not sampled and nor were those who declined to participate. People who had insight into their weaknesses may have been under-represented, thereby increasing the mean score in that group. Interestingly, no orthopaedic surgeons and two anaesthetists declined to participate.

我们的选择标准可能有偏差,因为休假整两周的医生没有被抽样,拒绝参与的医生也没有被抽样。了解自己弱点的人可能不愿意参加,从而提高了该组的平均得分。有趣的是,没有骨科医生拒绝参加,有两名麻醉师拒绝参加。

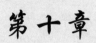

结论、致谢及参考文献的撰写

结论、致谢及参考文献部分是论文的末尾,也可算作论文的结束语。结论是正文的一部分,是对论文的最后总结,而致谢及参考文献虽然不是论文的正文内容,却是论文不可或缺的内容。要写就一篇优秀的骨科英文论文,写作者在研究中获得相关人员、机构的援手,以及参考大量文献是必不可少的,致谢及参考文献部分恰恰就是对此的说明。

10.1 结论

结论(conclusions)部分位于正文的最后,是整个论文的总论点,也是论文的重要组成部分,但并不是每篇研究论文都有单独的结论部分。一些期刊并没有严格要求论文要有结论部分,但即使没有这个要求,论文也至少应有1～2个段落起到结论部分的作用。通常来说,这样的段落会被包含在讨论部分中。结论的撰写并没有固定的模式,但不能完全重复前文内容,也不能仅仅叙述研究成果,而是需要对成果进行更加深入的评述。结论部分的撰写要求与摘要部分类似,但要避免完全重复摘要。结论的内容还可以包括指出研究成果的实际价值及提出展望,同时总结目前研究存在的问题及提出对今后研究的设想。

示 例

例 1

Conclusions

The findings from this large nationwide investigation do not support the hypothesis of a substantially beneficial effect of regional anesthesia compared with general anesthesia on all-cause mortality, but suggest that if a beneficial effect of regional anesthesia on postoperative mortality exists, it is likely to be more modest than previously reported. Additional research with studies powered to detect effect heterogeneity is needed to explore if specific population subgroups may meaningfully benefit from the use of regional anesthesia. Based on our data, the choice of anesthesia type should put emphasis on considerations other than differences in short-term mortality.

结论

这项全国性的大规模研究结果并不支持在各原因死亡率上,相对于全身麻醉,局部麻醉会有更有益的效果的假设,但是表明在术后死亡率上,如果局部麻醉的有益效果确实存在,则可能比之前报告的影响小。我们需要更多的研究来检测效果的异质性,以探索特定的亚群是否可以从局部麻醉的使用中获得好处。根据我们的数据,麻醉类型的选择应该把重点放在除短期死亡率的差异之外的考虑上。

[说明] 作为论文的结尾,此例结论部分不仅总结了论文的论点,还对以后的研究方向做出了推荐和预测。

例 2

Conclusions

The stereotypical image of male orthopaedic surgeons as strong but stupid is unjustified in comparison with their male anaesthetist counterparts. The comedic repertoire of the average anaesthetist needs to be revised in the light of these data. However, we would recommend caution in making fun of orthopaedic surgeons, as unwary anaesthetists may find themselves on the receiving end of a sharp and quick witted retort from their intellectually sharper friends or may be greeted with a crushing handshake at their next encounter.

结论

与男性麻醉师相比,男性骨科医生强壮但愚蠢的刻板印象是没有道理的。普通麻醉师需要根据这些数据修改自己的喜剧剧目。然而,我们建议在取笑骨科医生时要谨慎,因为自己可能会遭到更聪明的朋友们尖锐而机智的反驳,或者在下次见面时遇到他们的一个强有力的使骨头很痛的握手问候。

［说明］　作为文章末尾的结论句,是文章的核心句。此例的表达严谨不失幽默,用了一般现在时。

例3

Conclusions

Functional outcome after a nonoperatively treated type A spinal fracture is good, both at four as well as ten years post injury. Patients are only slightly disabled. For the group as a whole, four years after the fracture a steady state exists in functional outcome, which does not change systematically for at least ten years after the fracture. A small number of patients have a poor outcome, though none of our patients required surgery for late onset pain or late onset neurological deficit. Further research in this group of patients is advocated to reveal contributing factors.

结论

A型脊柱骨折非手术治疗后的功能结果良好,在伤后4年和伤后10年都是如此。患者都只有轻微残疾。总体来看,骨折后4年功能结果稳定,至少10年内不会发生系统性改变。尽管我们的患者中没有因迟发性疼痛或迟发性神经功能障碍而需要手术的,但也有一小部分患者的预后不佳。我们建议对这类患者做进一步研究,以揭示其原因。

［说明］　文献的最后一段用简洁的句子概括最终结论,同时也对将来进一步的研究提出了设想。

10.2　致谢

致谢(acknowledgements)是论文的附加部分,一般位于讨论和参考文献之间,但并非每篇论文都必须要有致谢部分。致谢是写作者对在研究或撰写过程中曾给予自己帮助的单位或个人表达谢意的段落。规范的致谢可以体现作者良好的科研素质。

致谢对象主要包括研究对象、参与部分研究工作但不具备作者署名资格的人、为研究提供便利的组织或个人、审阅或修改论文者、为研究提供资金资助的机构或个人等。需要注意的是,如果对提供资金的机构进行致谢,在提及资金来源时,应标注资金项目编号。写作者可以选择单独列出直接参与工作或提供帮助最大的人,对其他人可一并表示谢意。

致谢前应该征得被致谢人的同意。致谢中应该少说客套话,用简练的语言对主要帮助者表明谢意即可。例如,可用"The authors thank … for … ",而不用"The authors wish to thank … for …"这样的烦琐句式。

示 例

例 1

Acknowledgements

We thank … for his administrative support and … for technical support. We thank … for helpful advice and discussions. This work was supported by ….

致谢

我们感谢……的行政支持和……的技术支持。我们感谢……提供了有益的建议和讨论。这项工作得到了……的基金资助……

例 2

Acknowledgements

This work was part of the Program on … funded under the …, grant number is … Dr. ×××is a recipient of … The authors thank physicians, nurses, and research staff at … hospital for their assistance and support for this project.

致谢

这项工作是由……基金会资助的……项目,基金编号为……,……博士×××是……奖项的获得者。我们感谢……医院的医生、护士及研究人员对此研究的协助和支持。

10.3 参考文献

参考文献(references)是撰写论文时引用的相关资料,包括期刊、图书等。

参考文献的正确引用与否也是一篇论文质量是否合格的判定标准之一。引用参考文献的目的在于反映研究所借鉴内容的科研依据与科研基础,为读者判断研究的价值提供可靠依据。同时,通过著录他人的相关研究成果,写作者也是对他人的成果及著作权表示认同与尊重。因此,参考文献的质量影响论文的质量,写作者必须学会正确引用及著录参考文献。

(1)参考文献的引用原则

参考文献的引用原则包括以下几点:

① 选择较新的文献,避免引用过于陈旧的文献,尽量选取在具有权威性及专业性的期刊上发表过的文献,以体现研究领域的最新进展。

② 引用原始文献,避免因二次引用而出现引用错误。这也有助于写作者更深入地了解相关研究的情况。

③ 尽量引用已公开发表过的文献,少引用尚未公开发表的文献,如学术会议报告等。

④ 要严格筛选文献,医学英文论文引用的参考文献一般在 20 ~ 40 篇最佳。

(2)著录格式

不同期刊对著录格式的要求不同,写作者应严格按照期刊的要求去撰写。

但一般来说,医学期刊的著录格式一般采用温哥华参考文献格式(Vancouver reference style)。作者的姓用全称,名用缩写;引用文献的作者为 3 人以下时,将他们全部列出,若超出 3 人,则只需列出前 3 人,在其后加"et al.",不同作者中间用","分隔。期刊名通用缩写形式。

示 例

例1

Rotenstein LS, Torre M, Ramos MA, et al. Prevalence of burnout among physicians: a systematic review. JAMA. 2018;320:1131 −1150.

例2

Tsugawa Y, Newhouse JP, Zaslavsky AM, et al. Physician age and outcomes in elderly patients in hospital in the US: observational study. BMJ. 2017;

357:j1797.

例3

Waterman BR, Owens BD, Davey S, et al. The epidemiology of ankle sprains in the United States. J Bone Joint Surg Am. 2010;92:2279 −2284.

例4

Braun BL. Effects of ankle sprain in a general clinic population 6 to 18 months after medical evaluation. Arch Fam Med. 1999;8:143 −148.

例5

Leininger RE, Knox CL, Comstock RD. Epidemiology of 1. 6 million pediatric soccer-related injuries presenting to US emergency departments from 1990 to 2003. Am J Sports Med. 2007;35:288 −293.

论文研读

文献链接

经典文献链接:https://doi. org/10.1007/s11999-016-4827-y

标题:Where are the women in orthopedic surgery?

词　汇

discrepancy	n. 差异,不一致,偏差
affinity	n. 亲近,亲和力;喜好,喜爱
resident	n. 居民;(旅店)房客;住院医师
demographic	n. 人口统计数据;(尤指特定年龄段的)人群
	adj. 人口的,人口统计学的
deterrent	n. 威慑(物);遏制力;妨碍物
	adj. 威慑的,遏制的
paucity	n. 缺乏,短缺;少数,少量
perception	n. 理解,看法,认识;感知,感觉;洞察力,认识能力
attrition rate	磨损率,损耗率;流失率

physical strength　体力

critical mass　临界质量：最早源于核物理学，原指维持核子反应所需的裂变材料质量，现引申出来意指当一个物质达到临界点后，会引起连锁反应，量变引起质变

评　析

本文标题"骨科的女性在哪里？"是一个完整的问句，虽然简单，但紧扣研究内容，能引发读者的好奇心，激发读者的阅读兴趣。

摘要部分属于经典的结构式摘要，主要从背景（background）、问题/目的（questions/purposes）、方法（methods）、结果（results）、讨论（conclusions）几个方面叙述。读者通过摘要可看出整篇文章的研究内容和研究层次。摘要应该结构严谨，语言简洁干练，客观表达研究内容及结果。每位论文作者都应利用摘要简洁地传达自己的研究，突出其中最重要的方面。

本文以通过电子邮件发送调查问卷的方式，从个人属性、经验/接触、工作/生活等三个方面入手，统计分析了女性骨科医生选择骨科的原因及阻碍其他女性从事骨科领域工作的因素；研究调查了 232 名露丝·杰克逊骨科学会（RJOS）的活跃会员、候选人及常驻会员。

这项研究对 RJOS 的所有成员开放（556 人），其中 42% 的成员做出了回应。大多数受访者是执业或退休会员（81%），19% 是现役学员。近一半的受访者来自中西部或东北部地区。调查对象中最常见的专业为手外科（24%）、普通骨科（20%）、小儿骨科（19%）和运动医学（15%）。大多数受访者在学术机构（42%）或医院（21%）中执业。2/3 的受访者表示每周在直接患者护理活动上花费 40～70 个小时。75% 的受访者认为自己处于一段忠诚的关系中，52% 的人有孩子。

对 232 名受访者进行调查的结果显示，女性选择骨科的最常见的原因是享受动手工作（71%）、职业满意度（54%）和智力激发（53%）。大多数女性骨科医生的选择主要受个人属性的影响。相对较少的人是因为受到导师制（27%）或在医学院毕业前接触肌肉骨骼医学（16%）的启发。

女性不选择骨科的最常见原因包括以下三个方面：工作/生活考虑、个人属性、经验或导师制。78% 的受访者认为骨科医生不能很好地平衡工作和生活，而 74% 的受访者认为做骨科医生需要很多的体力，70% 的受访者觉得自己

在医学院或更早的时候缺乏良好的指导。

与个人兴趣相比,早期接触骨科的影响力较小,只有43%的受访者在医学院或更早或积极的榜样中受到导师的强大影响。只有16%的人认为在医学院接触肌肉骨骼医学是前五大影响因素之一。与个人兴趣相比,导师制度发挥的作用也较小,超过21%的受访者表示他们的培训方案中只有一名女性住院医师。大多数人报告说在骨科临床(52%)、骨科研究(82%)和非骨科临床教育活动(70%)中有1名或没有女性教员。

本文的结论:目前相对较少的这部分女性从事骨科工作纯粹是因为她们个人对骨科本质上的喜爱,而缺乏榜样和对骨科早期的接触可能是从事骨科领域工作女性人数持续不足的重要原因。此外,认为女性选择做骨科医生而牺牲了优越的生活方式的观点是不准确的。改善导师制度,增加医学生早期接触骨科和骨科医生的机会,可能会吸引更多不同的医学生群体选择骨科。

本文的不足之处主要围绕调查样本是否具有代表性来写。此部分的具体内容如下:

This study has several limitations. First, the survey was limited to members of the RJOS, and the experiences and opinions of the members might not reflect those of all women orthopaedic surgeons. However, this is the largest group of women orthopaedic surgeons of which we are aware, and this group has the advantages of internal diversity including subspecialty, geographic location, age, years out of training, and practice environment. Whether the RJOS membership is reflective of women orthopaedic surgeons in general is a difficult question to answer with accuracy.

这项研究有几个局限性。首先,调查仅限于RJOS的成员,成员的经历和观点可能无法代表所有女性骨科医生。但是,这是我们所知道的最大的女性骨科医生群体,并且该群体具有内部多样性的优势,包括不同的专科、地理位置、年龄、受训年限和实践环境。RJOS的成员能否反映女性骨科医生的整体情况,是一个很难准确回答的问题。

Additionally, response bias within RJOS may have influenced this study's findings, because those RJOS members (58% of membership) who did not participate in the survey might have different views and opinions from the cohort of respondents.

此外,RJOS 成员内部的反应偏差可能影响了本研究的结果,因为那些没有参与调查的 RJOS 成员(58%)可能与受访者群体有不同的观点和意见。

Finally because all answers were obtained from women orthopaedic surgeons, the reasons why women might not choose orthopaedic surgery are drawn from perceptions of current orthopaedic surgeons, which may not be entirely valid.

最后,由于所有答案都是从女性骨科医生那里获得的,因此女性不选择骨科的原因是来自目前骨科医生的看法,这可能并不完全有效。

附录一 骨科期刊

Archives of Orthopaedic and Trauma Surgery

Arthroscopy：*The Journal of Arthroscopic and Related Surgery*

BONE

Clinical Biomechanics

Clinical Journal of Sport Medicine

Clinical Orthopaedics and Related Research

Current Orthopaedics

Der Orthopäde

European Spine Journal

Foot & Ankle International

Gait & Posture

Hand Clinics

Injury

International Orthopaedics

Joint Bone Spine

Journal of Biomechanics

Journal of Neurosurgery：*Spine*

Journal of Orthopaedic & Sports Physical Therapy

Journal of Orthopaedic Research

Journal of Orthopaedic Science

Journal of Orthopaedic Trauma

Journal of Pediatric Orthopaedics

Journal of Pediatric Orthopaedics B

Journal of Shoulder and Elbow Surgery

Journal of Spinal Disorders & Techniques

Orthopedic Clinics of North America

ORTHOPEDICS

Osteoarthritis and Cartilage

Physical Therapy

Spine

The American Journal of Sports Medicine

The Journal of Arthroplasty

The Journal of Bone and Joint Surgery：American Volume

The Journal of Bone and Joint Surgery：British Volume

The Journal of Hand Surgery：European Volume

The Journal of Hand Surgery

The Knee

附录二　常用骨科词汇

A

AO 微型钛金属板 A. O. titanium plate

艾伯斯-舍恩伯格病(石骨症) Albers-Schonberg disease

阿斯曼氏病 Assmann disease

阿托品 atropine

癌 cancer, carcinoma, tumo(u)r

矮小症(非侏儒) microsoma

矮型的 brachymorphic

按摩 massage

胺 amine

凹 fovea

凹陷, 压痕 impression, invagination

凹陷骨折 depressed fracture

B

8 字形绷带 figure-of-eight bandage

拔出, 抽出 extraction

拔出器, 提取器 extractor

拔管, 除管法 extubation

摆动前期 pre-swing

摆动中期 mid-swing

疤痕 scar

扳机指 trigger finger

瘢痕性挛缩 scar contracture

瘢痕挛缩骨 cicatrical contracture bone

板层骨 lamellar bone

板障骨(颅骨间松质骨) diploe

半表面关节成形术 hemisurface arthroplasty

半侧肢体骨骺发育不良 dysplasia epiphysealis hemimelica

半骶化 hemisacralization

半关节成形术 hemiarthroplasty

半晶质的 semicrystalline

半乳糖脑苷脂 galactocerebroside

半脱位 semiluxation, subluxation

半月板 meniscus, semilunar cartilage

半月板成形术 meniscoplasty

半月板的 meniscal

半月板股骨间的 meniscofemoral

半月板胫骨间的 meniscotibial

半月板囊撕裂 meniscocapsular tear

半月板囊肿 meniscus cyst, cyst of menisci

半月板软骨撕裂 torn meniscus cartilage

半月板撕裂 tears of menisci

半月板周部 parameniscus

棒球指骨折 baseball finger fracture

棒球肘 baseball elbow

保存时间 preservation time

保存质量 preservation quality

爆裂骨折 burst fracture

杯状关节成形术 cup arthroplasty

贝克囊肿(腘窝囊肿) Baker's cyst

背侧插入性节段不稳定 dorsal intercalary / intercalated segment instability

背侧的 dorsal

背腹侧的 dorsoventral

背内侧的 dorsomedial

背屈步态 dorsalflexion gait

背痛 backache

背外侧的 dorsolateral

贝内特骨折 Bennett fracture

本体感受 proprioception

本体感受性神经肌肉强化 proprioceptive neuromuscular facilitation

苯巴比妥 phenobarbital

绷带 bandage

绷带法 bandaging

绷带卷 bandage roller

鼻烟窝 snuff-box

闭合性不全 dysraphism

闭合性创伤 closed wound

闭合性骨折 closed fracture

闭合性软组织损伤 closed soft tissue injury

闭合性损伤 closed injury

臂丛神经麻痹 brachial plexus paralysis

臂丛神经牵拉损伤 brachial plexus traction injury

臂丛神经损伤 brachial plexus injury

臂过小者,细臂者 microbrachius

臂痛 brachialgia

臂腿的 brachiocrural

臂肘的 brachiocubital

边缘骨刺 marginal osteophyte

边缘骨折 marginal fracture

边缘外生骨疣 marginal exostosis

编织骨 woven bone

扁平髋 coxa plana

扁平颅底 platybasia

扁平手 manus plana

扁平椎 vertebra plane

扁平足 flat foot

变形性关节病 arthronosos deformans

变形性骨关节炎 osteitis deformans

变形性脊椎病 spondylosis deformans

标准普通钢板 standard conventional plate

表面高恶性骨肉瘤 high-grade surface osteosarcoma

表面置换关节成形术 surface replacement arthroplasty

髌骨成形术 patellar arthroplasty

髌骨骨折 patellar fracture

髌骨缺如 absent patella

髌骨软化症 patellar chondromalacia

髌后脂肪垫挛缩 retropatellar fat pad contracture

髌前滑囊炎 prepatellar bursitis

髌下滑囊炎 infrapatellar bursitis

并指(趾)畸形 syndactylia,syndactyly,acrosyndactylism

病理性半脱位 pathological subluxation

病理性骨折 pathological fracture

玻璃化 vitrification

玻璃样的,透明的 vitreous

剥离骨折 cleavage fracture

剥离器 detacher,dissector,stripper

剥脱骨折 flake fracture

剥脱性骨软骨炎 osteochondritis dissecans

搏动 pulsation

搏动性疼痛 pulsating pain

跛行 claudication

补体 complement

不动关节 synarthrosis

不连接（骨）nonunion

不全骨折 infraction

不全脊柱裂 partialis rachischisis

不全强直 partial tetanus

不全瘫痪 incomplete paralysis

不全性骨折 insufficiency fracture

不全性麻痹 incomplete paralysis, paresis

不死性 immortalization

不完全性骨折 incomplete fracture

不稳步态 unsteady gait

不稳定骨折 unstable fracture

不稳定脊柱损伤 unstable spine injury

不稳定性 instability

布朗病 Blount disease, tibia vara

布罗迪脓肿 Brodie abscess

步行周期 walking cycle

C

长骨骨折 long bone fracture

长管状骨釉质细胞瘤 admantinoma of long bone

长期保存 long-term preservation

长收肌破裂 long adductor muscle rupture

残留半脱位 residual subluxation

残余足跟马蹄畸形 residual heel equinus

残肢 stump

层流净化 laminar flow cleaning

插入的 intercalary

插入关节成形术 interposition arthroplasty

产伤 birth injury

产伤性骨折 birth fracture

产伤性麻醉 birth paralysis

颤动现象 jitter

肠系膜上动脉综合征 superior mesentery artery syndrome

肠源性关节炎 enteropathic arthritis

车撞骨折 bumper fracture

陈旧性骨折 old fracture

晨僵 morning stiffness

撑开棒 distraction rod

成骨不全 osteogenesis imperfecta

成骨细胞 osteoblast

成骨性肉瘤 osteogenic sarcoma

成骨性纤维瘤 osteogenic fibroma

成骨性转移瘤 osteoblastic metastasis

成骨诱导物 osteogenic inducter/agent

成骨肿瘤 bone-forming tumor

成横纹肌细胞瘤 rhabdomyoblastoma

成肌细胞瘤 myoblastoma

成脊索细胞瘤 chordoblastoma

成角骨折 angulated fracture

成角截骨关节成形 angulation resection arthroplasty

成人获得性扁平足 adult-acquired flatfoot

成人脊柱侧凸 adult scoliosis

成人早老综合征（维尔纳综合征）adult progeria, Werner's syndrome

成髓作用, 髓细胞生成 myelopoiesis

成纤维细胞 fibroblast

迟发性佝偻病 late rickets, rachitis tarda

迟发性截瘫 late onset paraplegia

迟发性麻痹 delayed palsy, tardy palsy

弛缓性不全麻痹 flaccid paresis

弛缓性麻痹 flaccid palsy, flaccid paralysis

迟缓性麻痹 flaccid paralysis

尺骨粗隆 ulnar tuberosity

尺骨冠状突骨折 fracture of ulnar coronoid process

尺骨茎突骨折 fracture of ulnar styloid process

尺骨鹰嘴骨折 ulnar olecranal fracture

尺腕半月板 ulnocarpal meniscus

齿状突骨折 dens fracture, fracture of dens, fracture of odontoid peg

耻骨成形术 pubioplasty

耻骨联合分离 separation of the public symphysis

耻骨炎 osteitis pubis

初级骨化中心 primary ossification center

初期关节成形术 primary arthroplasty

除骨质，骨质丧失 deossification

杵臼关节 enarthrodial joint, enarthrosis

杵状指 clubbed finger

触觉的 tactile

穿通管 perforating canal

疮，溃疡 sore

创伤 trauma

创伤后骨关节炎 post-traumatic osteoarthritis

创伤后骨萎缩 post-traumatic atrophy of bone

创伤后关节炎 post-traumatic arthritis

创伤后脊髓空洞症 post-traumatic syringo-myelia

创伤性滑囊炎 traumatic bursitis

创伤性寰枢椎不稳 traumatic atlantoaxial unstableness

创伤性颅内出血 traumatic intracranial hemorrhage

创伤性神经症 traumatic neurosis

创伤性枢椎滑脱 traumatic spondylolisthesis of the axis

创伤性癔症 hysterotraumatism

槌状指 mallet finger

锤状趾 hammer toe

次级骨化中心 secondary ossification center

粗面内质网 rough endoplasmic reticulum

D

打入器,冲击器 impactor

大粗隆滑囊炎 trochanteric bursitis

大块骨溶解 massive osteolysis

大理石骨病 marble bone disease

呆小病,克汀病 cretinism

代谢性骨病 metabolic bone disease

带锁髓内针 interlocking medullary nailing

单臂畸形 monobrachia

单侧髁骨折 hemicondylar fracture

单纯冷保存 simple cold storage

单发性骨软骨瘤 solitary osteochondroma

单发性骨髓瘤 solitary myeloma

单发性肌炎 monomyositis

单骨性骨纤维异样增殖症 monostotic fibrous dysplasia

单光子 γ 射线吸收法 single photon absorptiometry

单一性髁囊肿 solitary bone cyst

蛋白多糖 protein polysaccharides

等动性肌力测定法 isokinetic dynamometry

低磷性佝偻病 hypophosphatemic ricket

低能量创伤 low energy trauma

低症磷酸酶 hypophosphatasia

骶骨发育不全 sacral agenesis

骶骨翼螺钉 alar screw

骶管裂孔 sacral hiatus

骶髂关节炎 sacroiliitis

骶髂劳损 sacroiliac strain

骶尾部畸胎瘤 sacrococcygeal teratoma

第五腰椎骶化 sacralization of fifth lumber vertebra

电动骨锯 electric bone saw

电灼术 electrocautery

动静脉瘤 arteriovenous aneurysm

动静脉瘘 arteriovenous fistula

动力性加压接骨板 dynamic compression plate

动力性绞锁固定钉 dynamic locking nail

动力性髁部螺钉 dynamic condylar screw

动脉成形术 arterioplasty

动脉瘤成形术 aneurysmoplasty

动脉瘤样骨囊肿 aneurysmal bone cyst

冻结肩,五十肩 frozen shoulder

短期保存 short-term preservation

短指(趾)骨 brachyphalangia

对称性不稳定 symmetric instability

对掌肌(立)成形术 opponoplasty, opponens plasty

多巴胺 dopamine

多巴酚丁胺 dobutamine

多发性成骨不全 multiple dysostosis

多发性骨骺发育不良 multiple epiphyseal dysplasia

多发性骨肉瘤 multicentric osteosarcoma

多发性骨髓瘤 multiple myeloma

多发性骨折 multiple fracture

多发性硬化 multiple sclerosis

多器官功能衰竭 multiple organ failure

断裂 disruption

E

鹅步 goose gait

鹅颈畸形 swan neck deformity

鹅足滑囊炎 pesanserinus bursitis

恶性高热 malignant hyperthermia

恶性骨巨细胞瘤 malignant giant cell tumor of bone

恶性软骨母细胞瘤 malignant chondroblastoma

恶性体液性高钙血症 humoral hypercalcemia of malignancy

儿童股骨头骨骺缺血性坏死 Legg-Calve-Perthes disease

儿童关节疡 pedarthrocace

二倍体 diploid

二腹肌 digastric

二磷酸盐 diphosphonate

二期闭合 secondary closure

二指(趾)节症 diphalangia

F

发育性髋关节发育不良 developmental dysplasia of the hip

反复性脱位 recurrence dislocation

反跳 rebound

泛发性纤维瘤病 generalized fibromatosis

放射免疫分析 radioimmunoassay

放射痛 radiating pain

放射性骨坏死 osteoradionecrosis

放射性核素扫描 radionuclide scanning

放射性脑脊髓病 radiation myeloencephalopathy

放射性同位素扫描 radioisotope scanning

非创伤性关节疾病 nontraumatic joint disorder

非对称性不稳定 asymmetric instability

非角度稳定性钢板 non-angular stable plate

非限制性肩关节成形（置换）术 unconstrained shoulder arthroplasty

非自攻钉 nonself-tapping

肥大性肺性骨关节病 hypertrophic pulmonary osteoarthropathy

肥大性关节炎 hypertrophic arthritis

肥大性滑膜炎 hypertrophic synovitis

肥大性假关节 hypertrophic pseudoarthrosis

肥厚性瘢痕 hypertrophic scar

腓肠肌-比目鱼肌无力步态 gastrocnemius-sole-us gait

腓肠肌性马蹄足 gastrocnemius equinus

腓骨肌痉挛性扁平足 peroneal spastic flatfoot

腓总神经卡压综合征 common peroneal nerve entrapment syndrome

废用性萎缩 disuse atrophy

分裂手 cleft hand, split hand

分裂足 cleft foot, split foot

分离插入关节成形术 distraction interposition arthroplasty

风湿性多肌痛 polymyalgia rheumatica

风疹性关节炎 rubella arthritis

蜂窝组织炎 cellulitis, phlegmon

缝合夹 wound clip

缝合锚钉 suture anchor

跗关节痛风性关节炎 gouty arthritis of tarsal joints

跗中关节脱位 dislocation of midtarsal joint

跗舟骨骨折 fracture of tarsus and scaphoid

氟骨症 fluorosis of bone

浮髌试验 floating patella test

复合性粉碎性骨折 compound comminuted fracture

复合性骨折 compound fracture

副韧带断裂 collateral ligament rupture

复位关节成形术 reduction arthroplasty

G

改良前肩峰成形术 improved foreacromioplasty

钙化性肌腱炎 calcified depository myotenositis

感染性关节炎 infectious arthritis

感染性滑囊炎 infective bursitis

感染性腱鞘炎 infective tenosynovitis

干骺端 metaphysis

干骺端骨折 fracture of metaphysis

干骺部结核 metaphyseal tuberculosis

干骺端脓肿 metaphyseal abscess

干骺续连症 metaphyseal aclasia

干髓端成骨不全 metaphyseal dysostosis

干髓端发育异常 metaphyseal dysplasia

干燥综合征 sicca syndrome

钢丝环 wire loop

高尔夫球肘 golfer's elbow

高弓内翻足 cavovarus

高弓外翻足 cavovalgus

高弓仰趾外翻 cavocalcaneovalgus

高能量创伤 high-energy trauma

髂粗隆 iliac tuberosity

髂胫束粗隆 tuberosity for iliotibial tract

跟骨步态 calcaneal gait

跟骨高压症 high pressure symptom of calcaneus

跟骨骨刺 heel spur

跟骨骨折 fracture of calcaneus

跟骨骨骺炎 calcaneal apophysitis

跟骨后滑囊炎 retrocalcaneal bursitis

跟腱断裂 achilles tendon rupture，rupture of achilles tendon

跟腱炎 achilles tendonitis

跟痛症 heel pain

跟趾步态 heel-to-toe gait

功能性腿长不等 functional leg length inequality

肱二头肌长头腱断裂 rupture of long tendon of biceps brachii

肱骨近端锁定钢板 locking proximal humeral plate

肱骨髁上骨折 supracondylar fracture of humerus

肱骨内外上髁炎 internal and external humeral epicondylitis

肱骨三角肌粗隆 deltoid tuberosity of humerus

共济失调步态 ataxia gait

佝偻病性驼背 ricketic kyphosis

孤立性骨囊肿 solitary bone cyst，unicameral bone cyst

股骨发育不全 femoral hypoplasia

股骨近端交锁钉 proximal femoral interlocking nail

股骨颈穿针导航 femoral neck needle penetration navigation

股骨髁部骨折 femoral condylar fracture

股骨髁上骨折 supracondylar fracture of femur

股骨髁支持钢板 femoral condylar supporting plate

股骨头凹 fovea of femoral head

股骨头缺血性坏死 avascular necrosis of femoral head

股骨头无菌性坏死 aseptic necrosis of femoral head

股四头肌成形术 quadricepsplasty

股四头肌肌腱断裂 rupture of femoral quadriceps muscle

骨板 bone lamellae

骨成形术 osteoplasty

骨出血 osteorrhagia

骨穿刺 bone puncture

骨脆症 fragilitas ossium

骨单位 osteon

骨钉 bone peg

骨发育异常 osteodysplasty

骨干 diaphysis

骨干发育异常 diaphyseal dysplasia

骨骺闭合，骨骺生长停止 epiphyseal arrest，epiphyseal closure

骨骼系统 skeletal system

骨关节炎 osteoarthritis

骨化性肌炎 myositis ossificans

骨棘球虫幼病 skeleton edinococcosis

骨基质 bone matrix

骨间前神经综合征 anterior interroseous nerve syndrome

骨筋膜间隙综合征 osteofascial compartment syndrome

骨巨细胞瘤 giant cell tumor of bone

骨螺钉 bone screw

骨密度 bone density

骨密度测定 bone densitometry

骨膜 periosteum

骨膜剥离器 raspatory，raspatorium

骨膜刀 periosteotome

骨膜性骨 periosteal bone

骨囊肿 bone cyst

骨内板 endosteal lamella

骨内力 internal force

骨内膜 endosteum

骨盆测量法 pelvimetry

骨盆对线 pelvic alignment

骨盆倾斜 inclinatio pelvis

骨盆旋转 pelvic rotation

骨软化病 osteomalacia

骨闪烁测量 bone scintimetry

骨松质 spongy/cancellous bone

骨松质螺钉 cancellous screw

骨髓发育不良 epiphyseal dysplasia

骨髓 bone marrow

骨髓腔 bone medullary cavity

骨突病 apophyseopathy

骨外力 external force

骨细胞 osteocyte

骨先质细胞 osteoprogenitor

骨纤维软骨发育异常 fibrocartilaginous dysplasia of bone

骨纤维结构不良 osteofibrous dysplasia

骨小管 bone canaliculus

骨小梁 trabeculae

骨性联合 synostosis

骨硬化病 osteopetrosis

骨硬化性发育不良 dysosteosclerosis

骨质减少性疾病 osteopenic disease

骨肿瘤 bone tumor

骨转移瘤 metastatic tumor of bone

骨赘 osteophyte

骨赘病 osteophytosis

骨组织形态计量学 bone histomorphometry

钴铬钼锻造合金 wrought cobalt-chromium tungsten nickel alloy

固定位置的螺钉 positioning screw

关节 articulation,joint

关节凹 articular fovea

关节半月板 articular meniscus

关节半月板病 meniscopathy

关节表面骨软骨发育不良 epiarticular osteochondrodysplasia

关节病步态 arthrogenic gait

关节出血 arthrorrhagia

关节穿刺[术] arthrocentesis

关节动度测量法 arthrometry

关节镜的 arthroscopic

关节镜肩峰下减压 arthroscopic subacromial decompression

关节镜手术刨削刀 arthroscopic shaver

关节镜下磨削软骨成形术 arthroscopic abrasion chondroplasty

关节面 articular facet/surface

关节面成形术 resurfacing arthroplasty

关节面骨折 articular surface fracture

关节囊成形术 capsuloplasty

关节内骨折 intra-articular fracture

关节切开术 arthrotome

关节软骨 articular cartilage

关节软骨板 articular lamella

关节软骨钙化症 chondrocalcinosis articularis

关节软骨钙质沉着病 articular chondrocalcinosis

关节鼠,关节内游离体 joint mouse

关节松弛症 arthrochalasis

关节退行性病变 joint degeneration

关节盂成形术 glenoplasty

关节粘连脊椎炎 ankylosing spondylitis

关节支柱骨折 articular pillar fracture

关节周围骨折 periarticular fracture

过度活动型半月板 hypermobile meniscus

过度外展综合征 hyperabduction syndrome

H

哈弗氏管 haversian canal

哈弗氏骨 haversian bone

褐黄病 ochronosis

横行步态 crab gait

横韧带撕裂 rupture of transverse ligament, transverse ligament rupture

横突肋凹 transverse costal fovea

红斑性肢痛病 erthromelalgia

骺板 epiphyseal plate

骺软骨板 epiphyses plate

后内侧旋转不稳定 posteromedial rotatory instability

后入路关节盂成形术 posterior glenoplasty

后纵韧带骨化 ossification of posterior longitudinal ligament

厚皮性骨膜病 pachydermoperiostosis

弧型重建钢板 curved reconstructive plate

滑车凹 trochlear fovea

滑动钉 sliding nail

滑动加压钉 sliding compression screw

滑膜 synovial membrane

滑膜层 synovial layer

滑膜囊肿 bursal cyst

滑膜炎 synovitis

滑囊病 bursopathy

滑囊炎 bursal inflammation

滑脱 olisthesis, olisthe, olisthy

化脓性瘢痕 purulent scar

化脓性关节炎 pyogenic arthritis

化脓性滑膜炎 septic bursitis

化脓性脊椎炎 pyogenic spondylitis

踝 ankle, malleolus

踝剥脱性骨软骨炎 talar osteochondritis dissecans

踝部骨折 ankle fracture

踝部螺钉 malleolar screw

踝部扭伤 ankle sprain

踝管综合征 tarsal tunnel syndrome

踝内侧副韧带损伤 injury of medial collateral ligament

踝外侧副韧带损伤 injury of lateral collateral ligament

坏死 necrosis

坏疽 gangrene

环绕椎板钢丝 circum-laminar wire

环形步态 circumduction gait

寰枢椎半脱位 atlantoaxial subluxation

寰枕融合症 atlas assimilation, assimilation of atlas, occipitalization

寰枕关节脱位 atlanto-occipital dislocation

慌张步态 festinating gait

黄骨髓 yellow bone marrow

黄韧带骨化 ossification of yellow ligament

黄[色]瘤病 xanthomatosis

喙锁韧带粗隆 tuberosity for coracoclavicular ligament

喙突粗隆 coracoid tuberosity

混合性结缔组织病 mixed connective tissue disease

活动度 mobility

活体组织检查 biopsy

J

基板,基底膜 basal lamina

基底内凹,颅底陷入症 basilar invagination, basilar impression

机械性损伤 mechanical injury

肌层 muscular layer

肌成形术 myoplasty

肌断裂 muscle rupture,myorrhexis

肌风湿病,纤维组织炎 fibrositis

肌腱病 tendinopathy

肌腱成形术 myotenontoplasty

肌腱炎 myotenositis,tendinitis,tendonitis

肌肉动作电位 muscle action potential

肌肉萎缩症 muscular dystrophy

肌肉硬化症 muscle gelling

肌肉运动诱发电位 muscle motion evoked potential

肌炎 myositis,myitis

肌营养不良步态 dystrophic gait

肌运动单位动作电位 motor unit action potential

畸形性骨炎 osteitis deformans

急性创伤性关节血肿 acute traumatic hemarthrosis

急性骨髓炎 acute osteomyelitis

急性挥鞭损伤 acute whiplash injury

急性缺血性挛缩 acute ischemic contracture

急性血源性骨髓炎 acute hematogenous osteomyelitis

挤压综合征 crush syndrome

脊髓半侧横断综合征 Brown-Sequard syndrome

脊髓出血 myelapoplexy,myelorrhagia

脊髓灰质炎 poliomyelitis

脊髓积水空洞症 hydrosyringomyelia

脊髓脊膜膨出 myelomeningocele

脊髓空洞症 syringomyelia,myelosyringosis

脊髓腔造影 myelography

脊髓软化症 myelomalacia

脊髓神经根病 myeloradiculopathy

脊髓栓系综合征 tethered cord syndrome

脊髓型颈椎病 cervical spondylotic myelopathy

脊髓诱发电位 spinal evoked potential

脊髓圆锥综合征 conus medularis syndrome

脊索 notochord

脊柱棘球蚴病 spinal hydatid disease

脊柱跛行 spinal claudication

脊柱侧弯 scoliosis

脊柱的 spinal,rachial,rachidial,rachidian

脊柱弓状后凸 round kyphosis

脊柱骨赘病 spinal osteophytosis

脊柱后凸 kyphosis

脊柱角状后凸 angular kyphosis

脊柱神经管闭合不全 spinal dysraphism

脊柱狭窄 spinal stenosis

脊椎闭合不全 dysraphism

脊椎病,脊柱病 spondylopathy,spondylosis, rachiopathy

脊椎骨软骨病 vertebral osteochondrosis

脊椎滑脱症 spondylolisthesis

脊椎化脓性骨髓炎 pyogenic osteomyelitis of the vertebra

脊椎肋骨发育不全 spondylocostal dysostosis

脊椎压迫性骨折 compression fracture of the vertebrae

计算机导航 computer-navigation

记忆合金 memory alloy

继发性骨折 secondary fracture

继发性基底压迹 secondary basilar impression

加压棒,压迫棒 compression rod

加压钢板 compression plate

加压拉力螺钉 compression lag screw

加压髓内针 compression intramedullary nail

痂皮 crust

家族性低磷酸盐血症 familial hypophos-phatemia

家族性骨膨胀症 familial osteoectasia

夹板[固定] splint,splinting,splintage

甲－骨综合征 onycho-osteodysplasia

假恶性骨化性肌炎 pseudomalignant myositis ossificans

假关节 pseudoarthrosis

假基底内陷 pseudobasilar invagination

假体 prosthesis

假指成形术 phalangization

间隙 interspace

间歇性跛行 intermittent claudication

间质骨板 interstitial lamella

间质细胞 mesenchymal cell

肩峰成形术 acromioplasty

肩峰的 acromial

肩峰下滑囊炎 subacromial bursitis

肩关节前脱位 anterior shoulder dislocation

肩关节周围炎 periarthritis scapulohumeralis

肩胛髂骨发育不良 scapuloiliac dysostosis

肩手症候群 hand-shoulder/shoulder-hand syndrome

肩锁关节成形术 acromioclavicular arthro-plasty

肩锁关节脱位 acromioclavicular dislocation

肩袖完全撕裂 complete tear of tendinous cuff

肩撞击综合征 shoulder impingement syndrome

剪刀步态 scissors gait

剪力 shear force

剪应力 shear stress

腱成形术 tendon plasty

腱断裂 tendon rupture

腱膜刀 aponeurotome

腱鞘 tendinous sheath

腱鞘囊肿 ganglion cyst

腱周围炎,腱鞘炎 peritendinitis

降钙素 calcitonin

交叉腿步态 cross-legged gait

交感神经型颈椎病 sympathetic type of cervical spondylosis

交锁钉 interlocking nail

交替步态 reciprocating gait

焦磷酸钙沉积病 calcium pyrophosphate deposition disease

角化病 keratosis

角形钢板,角叶状钢板 angled blade plate

接骨板 blade plate

接骨点炎 enthesitis

接骨术 osteosynthesis

节段 segment

节段性穿钢丝 segmental wiring

结缔组织按摩 connective tissue massage

结核 tuberculosis

结核性滑囊炎 tuberculous synovitis

结核性脊椎炎 tuberculous spondylitis

结节病 sarcoidosis

截骨术 osteotomy

截肢术 amputation

截肢端成形术 amputation stump plasty

解剖刀,手术刀 scalpel

解剖颈骨折 fracture of anatomic neck

解剖型钢板 anatomic plate

筋膜病 fasciopathy

筋膜成形术 fascioplasty

筋膜刀 fasciotome

筋膜间隔综合征 fascial compartment syndrome

紧张性手足徐动症 tension athetosis

进行性神经性肌萎缩(夏科-马里-图斯病) Charcot-Marie-Tooth disease

近位指骨短小症 brachybasophalangia

浸润 infiltration

经皮微创钢板 minimally invasive percutaneous plate

经皮椎体成形术 percutaneous vertebroplasty

颈臂丛综合征 cervicobrachial syndrome

颈肋综合征 cervical rib syndrome

颈颅综合征 cervicocranial syndrome

颈围领 neck band

颈椎病 cervical spondylosis

颈椎病性肌萎缩 cervical spondylotic amyotrophy

颈椎带锁型钢板 cervical spine locking plate

颈椎后韧带断裂 rupture of posterior ligament of cervical spine

颈椎滑脱 cervical spondylolisthesis

颈椎间盘突出症 cervical disc herniation

颈椎椎板双侧开门成形术 bilateral expansive laminoplasty of cervical vertebra

胫侧半肢畸形 tibial hemimelia

胫骨平台骨折 tibial plateau fracture

胫前间室综合征 anterior tibial compartment syndrome

痉挛性步态 spastic gait

痉挛性斜颈 spasmodic torticollis

静脉曲张病 varicosis

局部退行性椎间盘病 localized degenerative disc disease

局灶性蛛网膜瘢痕形成 local arachnoid scarring

矩形钉 rectangle nail

巨臂 macrobrachia

巨人症 gigantism

距腓前韧带断裂 rupture of anterior talofibular ligament

距骨撕脱骨折 talar avulsion fracture

距骨周围脱位 peritalar dislocation

绝经妇女骨质疏松症 postmenopausal osteoporosis

K

髋关节炎 arthritis of the hip

髋关节和膝关节置换手 hip and knee joint replacement

髁部骨折 condylar fracture

髁间 T 形骨折 intercondylar T fracture

髁间 Y 形骨折 intercondylar Y fracture

髁接骨板 condylar plate

可动关节 diarthrosis

可吸收缝合线 absorbable suture

可吸收螺钉 bioabsorbable screw

可拽出钢丝 pull-out wire

空心螺钉 cannulated screw

跨阈步态(鸡步)steppage gait

髋部骨折 hip fracture

髋关节 hip joint

矿质化 mineralization

扩髓钉 reamed nail

L

拉力,拉伸 tension

劳损 strain

老年性骨质疏松症 senile osteoporosis

老年性强直性脊柱骨增殖症 senile ankylosing hyperostosis

老年性驼背 senile kyphosis

肋骨骨折 fracture of rib

肋软骨炎 costal chondritis, costochondritis

肋锁综合征 costoclavicular syndrome

肋椎角差异 rib vertebral angle difference

泪珠状骨折 teardrop fracture

类半月板 meniscus homologue

类风湿性关节炎 rheumatoid arthritis

类肉瘤病,结节病 sarcoidosis

类肢端肥大症 acromegaloidism

梨状肌综合征 piriformis syndrome

立行不能 astasia-abasia

连枷关节 flail joint

连枷指 flail digit

连枷足 flail foot

连续缝合 continuous suture

淋病性足跟痛 gonorrheal heel

淋球菌性关节炎 gonococcal septic arthritis

磷酸酯 acidic phospholipid

流行性肌炎 epidemic myositis

瘤样病变 tumor-like lesion

六指畸形 hexadactyly

漏斗胸 funnel breast, pectus excavatum

颅底凹陷,扁颅底 basilar impression

颅底骨折 fracture of skull base

颅骨面骨发育不全 cranio facial dysostosis

颅骨软化 craniotabes

轮替运动不能 adiadochokinesis

螺丝刀 screwdriver

螺纹钢棒 threaded rod

麻痹 palsy, paralysis, paresis

麻痹步态 paralytic gait

麻醉 narcosis, anesthesia

M

马蹄内翻足 equinovarus, talipes equinovarus

马蹄外翻足 talipes equinovalgus

马蹄足步态 equinus gait

马尾性跛行 cauda equina claudication

马尾综合征 cauda equina syndrome

慢性骨髓炎 chronic osteomyelitis

慢性局限性骨脓肿 localized bone abscess

梅毒性骨炎 osteitis syphilitica

梅毒性关节炎 syphilitic arthritis

梅毒性滑囊炎 luetic bursitis

梅花钉 plum blossom nail

孟氏骨折 Monteggia fracture

弥漫性特发性骨肥大症 diffuse idiopathic skeletal hyperostosis

弥漫性血管内凝血 disseminated intravascular coagulation

密质骨 compact bone

摩擦性尺神经炎 friction neuritis of ulnar nerve

摩擦性腱鞘炎 crepitant friction tenosynovitis

莫顿跖骨痛 Morton metatarsalgia

末端病 enthesopathy

末节指(趾)骨粗隆 tuberosity of distal phalanx

末节指骨短小症 brachytelephalangia

膜内成骨 intramembranous ossification

拇趾僵直 hallux rigidus

拇趾外翻 hallux valgus

拇趾滑囊炎 bunion

拇趾内翻 hallux varus

膜状管 membranous tube

N

难治性佝偻病 refractory rickets

难治性疼痛,顽固性疼痛 intractable pain

囊 bursa,sac,capsule,capsul

囊内骨折 intracapsular fracture

囊外骨折 extracapsular fracture

囊性脊柱裂 spinal bifida cystica

囊性血管瘤病 cystic angiomatosis

内八字步态 toe-in gait

内侧半月板 medial meniscus

内侧的 medial

内侧胫骨粗隆 medial tibial tuberosity

内翻 inversion,varus

内反应力 internal reaction force

内固定问题研究学会 association for the study of problem of intenal fixation

内环骨板 inner circumferential lamellae

内皮层 endothelium layer

内生软骨瘤病,Ollier 病 enchondromatosis, Olliser disease

内收型骨折 adduction fracture

内紊乱症 internal derangement

内应力 internal stress

黏多糖 glycosaminoglycan

黏液瘤 myxoma

黏液囊肿 mucocele

碾挫骨折 crush fracture

碾挫综合征 crush syndrome

尿毒症性骨营养不良 uraemic osteodystrophy

尿黑酸尿性关节炎 alcaptonuric arthritis

凝血 blood coagulation

牛皮癣性关节炎 psoriatic arthritis

扭转(转动)torsion

扭转骨折 torsional fracture

扭转力 torsional force

纽扣缝合 button suture

脓血症,脓毒症 pyemia

脓肿 abscess

P

帕金森步态 Parkinsonian gait

盘状半月板 discoid meniscus

盘状外侧半月板 discoid lateral meniscus

蹒跚步态(鸭步)waddling gait

蹒跚步态(与酒精中毒有关)staggering gait,reeling gait

旁弯骨折 greenstick fracture

跑步者膝盖 runner's knee

盆骨 pelvic bone

膨胀式带锁加压钉 interlocking expanding compressive screw

皮层诱发电位 cerebral evoked potential

皮肤划纹症 dermatographism

皮肌炎 dermatomyositis

皮内缝合 subcuticular suture

皮下气肿 aerodermectasia

皮样囊肿 dermoid cyst

皮质骨螺钉 cortical bone screw

皮脂腺囊肿,粉瘤 sebaceous cyst

疲劳骨折 fatigue fracture,stress fracture

疲劳极限 fatigue limit

疲劳试验 fatigue test

疲劳寿命 fatigue life

偏瘫步态,半身不遂步态 hemiplegic gait

偏臀步态 gluteal gait

平背 flat back,poker back

平衡 equilibrium,balance

平衡钢板 neutralizing plate

平足,扁平足 flatfoot

破骨细胞 osteoclast

Q

起立不能 astasia

髂耻滑囊炎 iliopectineal bursitis

髂骨骨髓炎 osteomyelitis of the ilium

髂骨致密性骨炎 osteitis condensans ilium

髂窝脓肿 iliac abscess

髂腰韧带试验 iliolumbar ligament test

牵伸 stretch

前臂 antebrachium,forearm,lower arm

前臂间室综合征 forearm compartment syndrome

前臂加压试验 forearm compression test

前抽屉试验 anterior drawer test

前后抽屉试验 anterior-posterior drawer test

前进试验 march test

前列腺素 prostaglandin

前路钢板 anterior plate

前内侧旋转不稳定 anteromedial rotatory instability

前屈试验 forward bending test

前置术,前移术 advancement

前纵韧带骨化 ossification of the anterior longitudinal ligament

强直 rigidity,stiffness,ton-,tono

强直性脊柱炎 ankylosing spondylitis

强直性痉挛 titanic contraction

羟基磷灰石 hydroxyapatite

羟基磷灰石沉积病 hydroxyapatite deposition disease

桥接钢板 bridging plate

切迹 incisure

切开复位术 open reduction

切口 incision

琴键试验 piano key test

青春期髋内翻,股骨头骨骺滑脱症 coax vara adolescentium

青少年脊柱后凸 adolescent kyphosis

青少年特发性脊柱侧弯 adolescent idiopathic scoliosis

轻弹试验 flip test

清创术 debridement

屈曲 flexion

躯干前屈症 bent back,camptocormia

全身骨发育不全 general dysostosis

全身纤维性骨炎 osteitis fibrosa generalisata

拳击手骨折 boxer's fracture

拳击肘 boxer's elbow

缺血性骨不连 avascular nonunion

缺血性坏死 avascular necrosis,ischemic necrosis

缺血性挛缩 ischemic contracture

R

桡神经卡压综合征 radial sensory nerve entrapment syndrome

桡尺骨融合 radioulnar synostosis

桡侧半肢畸形 radial hemimelia

桡骨茎突骨折,驾驶员骨折 radial styloid fracture,chauffeur's fracture

桡骨头半脱位,牵引肘 Malgaigne's luxation

桡骨小头半脱位 radial head subluxation

人体人字形绷带 body spica

韧带 ligament

韧带联合 syndesmosis

绒毛结节性滑膜炎 villonodular synovitis

溶解 dissolution

融合 fusion,coalition,-desis

肉瘤 sarcoma

褥疮 bedsore,pressure sore

褥式缝合 mattress suture

软骨化中心 chondrification center

软骨刀 ecchondrotome

软骨发育不全症 achondroplastic dwarfism

软骨钙质沉着病,软骨钙化症 chondrocalci-nosis

软骨结合 synchondrosis

软骨瘤 chondroma

软骨黏液样纤维瘤 chondromyxoid fibroma

软骨母细胞 chondroblast

软骨内成骨 endochondral ossification

软骨内骨发育不全 enchondral dysostosis

软骨肉瘤 chondrosarcoma

软骨软化 chondromalacia

软骨退行性变 cartilaginous degeneration

软骨炎 chondritis

软骨营养不良 chondrodystrophia,chondro-dystrophy

软骨游离体 cartilaginous loose body

S

三角凹 triangular fovea

三角肌粗隆 deltoid tuberosity

三角肌挛缩 deltoid contracture

三翼钉 Smith-Petersen nail

色素性绒毛结节性滑膜炎 pigmented villon-dular synovitis

纱布绷带 gauze bandage

上臂 upper limb,upper extremity,upper arm

上臂外侧 lateral arm

上皮层 epithelial layer

神经丛病 plexopathy

神经丛病损 neuroplexic lesion

神经根病变 radiculopathy

神经根型颈椎病 cervical spondylotic radicu-lopathy

神经节 ganglion

神经卡压综合征 nerve entrapment syndrome

神经瘤 neuroma

神经嵌压症 entrapment neuropathy

神经鞘瘤病 neurinomatosis

神经鞘脂贮积症 sphingolipidosis

神经切断术 neurotomy

神经疼痛性肌萎缩症 neuralgic amyotrophy

神经性关节功能障碍 neuroarticular dysfunction

神经炎 neuritis

神经源性跛行 neurogenic claudication

肾性侏儒[症] renal dwarfism

肾性骨病变 renal osteodystrophy

生物力学 biomechanics

生长板 growth plate

失调步态 incoordinated gait

石膏绷带 plaster bandage

石膏症,大理石骨 osteopetrosis

食指拇指化 pollicization of index finger

蚀化性关节炎 erosion arthritis

匙状钢板 spoon plate

匙状手 spoon hand

手部腱鞘滑膜炎 tenosynoritis of the hand

手法复位 manipulative reduction,manual reduction

手骨折 hand fracture

手术 operation, surgery, procedure

手术复位 surgical reduction

手掌腱膜挛缩症 dupuytren contracture

手指屈肌腱鞘炎 tenosynovitis of hand flexor tendon

手足搐搦 tetany

手足徐动症,指痉症 athetosis

受体 receptor

受限 limitation

枢椎齿状突骨折 odontoid fracture of the axis

衰弱背 failed back

栓塞 embolism

双[散]人字绷带 double spica

双层冷冻保存 two-layer cold storage

双踝骨折 bimalleolar ankle fracture, bicondylar fracture

双髋石膏绷带 double hip plaster bandage, double hip spica

双足行走 bipedal walking

水肿 edema

撕脱骨折 avulsion fracture

四甲基乙二胺 tetramethyl ethylene diamine

四肢瘫 tetraplegia

松弛 laxity, relaxation, chalasia

松质骨螺钉 cancellous bone screw

髋关节真菌病 coxarthrocace

髓内棒 intramedullary rod

髓内钉 intramedullary nail

髓内针 intramedullary pin

髓屈步态(见于腓神经麻痹)equinus gait

T

钛 titanium

瘫痪性脊柱后凸 paralytic kyphosis

弹响肩 snapping shoulder

弹响髋 snapping hip

弹性绷带 elastic bandage

弹性模量 elastic modulus

弹性髓内针 flexible medullary nail

碳素接骨板 carbon plate

体感诱发电位 somatosensory evoked potential

痛性步态,防痛步态 antalgic gait

骰骨骨折 fracture of cuboid

腿、踝或脚肿胀 swollen legs, ankles, or feet

腿长不等 leg length inequality

退行性椎间盘病变 degenerative disc disease

臀大肌步态(见于臀大肌麻痹)gluteus maximus gait

臀肌粗隆 gluteal tuberosity

拖行步态 shuffling gait

拖拉步态 drag gait

脱位 dislocation, dearticulation, luxation

跖筋膜炎 plantar fasciitis

W

外翻缝合 everting suture

外环骨板层 outer circumferential lamellae

外展 abduction

外展步态 abduction gait

外展倾斜步态 abductor lurch/inclined gait

弯曲 bending, curvature, curve

弯曲(异常)gryposis

腕尺管综合征 ulnar tunnel syndrome

腕骨背伸不稳定 dorsal intercalated segment instability

腕骨掌屈不稳定 volar intercalated segment instability

腕管综合征 carpal tunnel syndrome

腕下垂 carpoptosis, wristdrop

网球肘 tennis elbow

维生素过多症 hypervitaminosis

维生素缺乏症 avitaminosis

萎缩 atrophy

无臂 abrachia

无汗症 anhidrosis

无机焦磷酸 inorganic pyrophosphate

无菌性坏死 aseptic necrosis

无髓神经纤维 unmyelinated nerve fiber

舞蹈病 chorea

舞蹈步态 dancing gait

X

膝关节炎 knee arthritis

膝关节痛 knee joint pain

膝关节置换术 knee joint replacement

膝后十字韧带损伤 injury of posterior cruciate ligament of knee

膝劳损、退化与关节炎 knee injury, degeneration & arthritis

膝内侧副韧带损伤 injury of lateral collateral ligament of knee

膝前十字韧带损伤 injury of anterior cruciate ligament of knee

膝韧带撕裂 knee torn ligaments

系统疾病 systemic disease

细臂,臂过小 microbrachia

峡部不连,峡部裂 spondylolysis

狭窄 stenosis

狭窄性腱鞘炎 stenosing tenosynovitis

下背部 low back

下肢不等长 leg length discrepancy

先天性扁平足 congenital flatfoot

先天性副肌强直 congenital paramyotonia

先天性高位肩胛 congenital high scapula

先天性胫骨假关节 congenital tibial pseudarthrosis

先天性髋关节脱位 congenital dislocation of hip

先天性髋内翻 congenital coxa varus

先天性马蹄内翻足 congenital talipes equinovalgus

行军性骨折 march fracture

纤维瘢痕 fibrous scar

纤维化,纤维变性 fibrosis

纤维瘤 fibroma

纤维脂肪瘤病 fibrolipomatosis

纤维组织肌痛 fibromyalgia

显性脊柱裂 overt spinal dysraphism

线状瘢痕 linear scar

腺病(腺肿大,尤指淋巴结肿大) adenopathy

箱式缝合 box suture

小脑病步态,摇摆步态 cerebellar gait

小腿抽筋 leg cramp

小腿弯曲症 crus antecurvatus

协同不能 asynergia

胸骨穿刺 sternal puncture

胸廓出口综合征 thoracic outlet syndrome

胸腔穿刺术 thoracentesis

胸椎管狭窄征 thoracic spinal stenosis

胸椎间盘病变 thoracic disc disease

胸椎后纵韧带骨化 thoracic ossification of posterior longitudinal ligament

休门氏症 Scheuermann's disease

悬吊术 suspension

旋前肌粗隆 pronator tuberosity

旋前圆肌综合征 pronator syndrome

旋转不稳定 rotatory instability

旋转肌袖损伤 rotator cuff injury

血窦 sinusoid

血管病 vasculopathy

血管瘤病 angiomatosis

血钾过少,低钾血症 hypopotassemia

Y

腰椎间盘突出症 lumbar disc herniation

压力/加压绷带 compression/pressure bandage

压应力 compressive stress

延迟的首次性伤口闭合 delayed primary closure

延迟缝合 delayed suture

延迟性成骨不全,骨脆症 osteopsathyrosis, tardy imperfect osteogenesis

延髓空洞症 syringobulbia

腰骶不稳定 lumbosacral instability

腰椎穿刺 lumbar puncture

腰椎间盘疾病 lumbar disc disease

腰椎间盘突出 lumbar herniated disc

一期闭合 primary closure

一期缝合 primary suture

移植物抗宿主病 graft versus host disease

异位,错位 dystopia,ectopia,ectopy

易疲劳材料 fatigueprone material

隐性脊柱闭合不全,脊柱隐裂 occult spinal dysraphism

鹰嘴部滑囊炎 olecranal bursitis

应力 stress

应力保护 stress protection

应力保护性骨萎缩 stress protection atrophy

应力骨折 stress fracture

应力集中 stress concentration

应用透视导航 fluoro-navigation

应力线 stress line

硬化 sclerosis

硬化性骨髓炎 sclerosing osteomyelitis

硬膜穿刺 dural puncture

尤因肉瘤 Ewing's sarcoma

有髓神经纤维 myelinated nerve fiber

诱发电位 evoked potential

原发性骨质疏松症 primary osteoporosis

原发性基底压迹 primary basilar impression

原位成骨 appositional bone formation

圆背 round back

圆刀 round-edged knife

远近端再对线 proximal and distal realignment

月骨周围不稳定 perilunate instability

运动失灵,运动不能 akinesia

运动诱发电位 motor evoked potential

运用不能(指精神性上的) apraxia

Z

再对线 realignment

早发性大理石骨病 osteopetrosis with precocious manifestations

早老症 progeria,premature senility

早熟性闭合 premature closure

粘连性瘢痕 adherent scar

张力带 tension band

张力带钢丝,张力性钢丝带 tension band wiring

张力带固定 tension band fixation

张应力 tensile stress

跖骨骨折 fracture of metatarsal bone

跖跗关节脱位 dislocation of tarsometatarsal

joint

爪状趾 claw toe

阵挛 clonus

肢端骨发育不全 acrodysostosis

肢端缺氧症,肢端假死症 acroasphyxia

脂肪脊髓脊膜膨出 lipomyelomeningocele

脂肪栓塞综合征 fat embolism syndrome

脂质 lipids

直视复位 euthyphoria reduction, reduction under direct visualization

跖骨粗隆 tuberosity of metatarsal bone

跖骨头骨软骨炎 osteochondritis of metatarsal head

指(趾)骨缺少 hypophalangism

指(趾)甲过小[症] micronychia

指(趾)节减少症 hypophalange

指压痕 digital impression

趾骨骨折 toe fracture

治疗性按摩 therapeutic massage

致密性成骨发育不全症 pyknodysostosis, pycnodysostosis

踵趾步态 tandem gait

中位指骨短小症 brachymesophalangia

中央脊髓综合征 central cord syndrome

中央静脉窦 central venous sinus

周围血管疾病 peripheral vascular disease

轴向力 axial force

肘管综合征 cubital tunnel syndrome

舟骨粗隆 tuberosity of navicular bone

拄杖行走 crutch walking

注射 injection

椎板 vertebral lamina

椎弓板 lamina of vertebral arch

椎弓根节段性差异 segmental difference of pedicle of vertebral arch

椎骨刀,脊柱刀 rachitome

椎管穿刺法 rachicentesis, rachiocentests

椎管闭合不全 spinal dysraphism

椎管内出血 intraspinal hemorrhage, hematorrhachis

椎间盘 intervertebral disc

椎间盘后凸 herniated disk

椎间盘内裂症 internal disc disruption

椎间盘内瘢痕形成 intradiscal scarring

椎前层 prevertebral layer

姿势性对线 postural alignment

姿势性圆背 postural round back

自攻螺丝 self tapping screw

自身加压接骨板 self compressing plate

自身免疫病 autoimmune disease

足病,脚病 pedopathy

足部骨折 foot fracture

足穿通症 pedal perforation disease

足溃疡 foot ulcer

足跟步态 heel gait

足尖步态,趾步 toe gait

足尖向内步态 in-toeing gait

足尖向外步态 out-toeing gait

足下垂步态 foot-drop gait

组织细胞增多症 histiocytosis

坐骨结节滑囊炎 ischiogluteal bursitis

坐骨神经痛 sciatica

佐剂性关节炎 adjuvant arthritis

参考文献

Anderson ML, Lu FW, Yang J. Physical activity and weight following car ownership in Beijing, China:quasi-experimental cross sectional study. BMJ. 2019;367:l6491.

Brison RJ, Day AJ, Pelland L, et al. Effect of early supervised physiotherapy on recovery from acute ankle sprain:randomised controlled trial. BMJ. 2016;355:i5650.

Elsharkawy A, Ali AM. Clinical outcome of Decompressive Craniectomy operation for the management of acute traumatic brain injury. OJMN. 2019;9(3):281 – 291.

Emelifeonwu JA, Hazelwood JE, Nolan O, et al. Bend it like Beckham or fix them like Florence-proportional representation of healthcare in New Year honours:an observational study. BMJ. 2019;367:l6721.

Frobell RB, Roos HP, Roos EM, et al. Treatment for acute anterior cruciate ligament tear: five-year outcome of randomised trial. BMJ. 2013;346:f232.

Goldberg Y, Danckert J. Traumatic brain Injury, boredom and depression. Behav. Sci (Basel). 2013;3(3):434 – 444.

Grey A, Bolland MJ, Dalbeth N, et al. We read spam a lot:prospective cohort study of unsolicited and unwanted academic invitations. BMJ . 2016;355:i5383.

Guo JJ, Tang N, Yang HL. Impact of surgical approach on postoperative heterotopic ossification and avascular necrosis in femoral head fractures: a systematic review. International Orthopaedics (SICOT). 2010;34:319 – 322.

Guo JJ, LukKDK , Karppinen J, et al. Prevalence, distribution, and morphology of ossification of the ligamentum flavum:a population study of one thousand seven hundred thirty-six magnetic resonance imaging scans. SPINE. 2010;35(1):51 – 56.

Jong MBD, Houwert RM, Heerde SV, et al. Surgical treatment of rib fracture nonunion: a single center experience. Injury. 2018;49(3):599 – 603.

Koplewitz G, Blumenthal DM, Gross N, et al. Golf habits among physicians and surgeons:observational cohort study. BMJ. 2018;363:k4859.

Li JF, Luo LQ. Nurturing undergraduate researchers in biomedical sciences. Cell. 2020;182:1 – 4.

Patorno E, Neuman MD, Schneeweiss S, et al. Comparative safety of anesthetic type for hip fracture surgery in adults: retrospective cohort study. BMJ. 2014; 348: g4022.

Post RB, van der Sluis CK, Leferink VJM, et al. Nonoperatively treated type A spinal fractures: mid-term versus long-term functional outcome. International Orthopedics (SICOT). 2009; 33: 1055 – 1060.

Rohde RS, Wolf JM, Adams JE. Where are the women in orthopedic surgery? Clin Orthop Relat Res. 2016; 474: 1950 – 1956.

Rizvi SMT, Bishop M, Lam PH, et al. Factors predicting frequency and severity of post-operative pain after arthroscopic rotator cuff repair surgery. AM J SPORT MED. 2020; DOI: 10. 1177/0363546520971749.

Samuelsen BT, Desai VS, Turner NS, et al. Generational differences in grit, self-control, and conscientiousness among orthopaedic surgeons from millennials to baby boomers. J Bone Joint Surg Am. 2019; 101: e71(1 – 8).

Subramanian P, Kantharuban S, Subramanian V. Orthopaedic surgeons: as strong as an ox and almost twice as clever? Multicentre prospective comparative study. BMJ. 2011; 343: d7506.

Vasta S, PapaliaR, Albo E, et al. Top orthopedic sports medicine procedures. JOSR. 2018; 13: 190.

Wallis CJD, Ravi B, Coburn N, et al. Comparison of postoperative outcomes among patients treated by male and female surgeons: a population based matched cohort study. BMJ. 2017; 359: j4366.

Xu YJ, Wu KL, Guo JJ. Comparison of clinical and patient-reported outcomes of three procedures for recurrent anterior shoulder instability: anthroscopic Bankart repair, capsular shift, and open Latarjet. JOSR. 2019; 14: 326.

Zimerman A, Worsham C, Woo J, et al. The need for speed: observational study of physician driving behaviors. BMJ. 2019; 367: l6354.